The Elements of Chemistry A Comprehensive Guide

Johnathan Miller

Copyright © [2023]

Author: Johnathan Miller

Title: The Elements of Chemistry A Comprehensive Guide

All rights reserved. Chromium Treatment from Contaminated Soil and Groundwater No part of this publication may be reproduced, stored in a retrieval system, or transmitted, in any form or by any means, electronic, mechanical, photocopying, recording, or otherwise, without the prior written permission of the publisher or author.

This book was printed and published by in [2023].

ISBN:

Table of content

Chapter name	Page No
1. Chemical Principles: An Overview	1
2. The Structure of Atoms	29
3. Periodic Table	42
4. To bond chemically	53
5. Involvement in Reactions	62
6. Bases and Acids	71
7. Thermodynamics in Chemistry	82
8. Synthetic Organic Chemistry	93
9. A Brief Introduction to Inorganic Chemistry	105
10. Laboratory Methods and Analytical Chemistry	11

Chapter 1:
Chemical Principles: An Overview

1.1   What is Chemistry?

Simply put, what is chemistry?

Chemistry is the study of matter and its interactions, including its make-up, structure, and behaviour. Because it bridges the gap between physics and biology and sheds light on the behaviour of matter at the atomic and molecular levels, chemistry is frequently referred to as the central science. Everything from the food we eat to the medicines we take and the materials we use have some connection to chemistry, which plays a key role in our knowledge of the natural world.

Organic chemistry, inorganic chemistry, physical chemistry, analytical chemistry, and biochemistry are just a few of the many subfields that fall under the umbrella of "chemistry." Each of these subfields investigates a unique facet of matter's metamorphoses. Learning about chemistry's foundations, principles, and potential uses is essential to grasping the field's relevance.

In this in-depth investigation, we will go through chemistry's evolution, delve into the underlying principles that support this science, investigate chemistry's many subfields and their practical applications, and speculate on the field's opportunities and threats in the twenty-first century. This in-depth analysis will help you better comprehend what chemistry is and how it influences our daily lives.

Annotated Contents

1. Introduction
- Why Chemistry Is So Vital
- The Topics We Will Cover

2. An Outline of Chemical Development
- Deep History
The Evolution from Alchemy to Contemporary Chemistry
The Age of Chemical Progression
Significant Developments in the 19th and 20th Centuries
Modern Chemical Processes

3. An Introduction to Chemistry
Elements and Atoms
Intermolecular Forces
Reactions in the Laboratory
"The Periodic Table"
Stoichiometry and Chemical Equations

4. Science of Organic Compounds
Organic Substances
Carbon-Hydrogen Bonds
- Categories of Use
Definition of Isomerism
Mechanisms of Reaction

5. Science of Inorganic Substances
Inorganic Substances
Synthetic Coordination Compounds
Metals in Transition
- Metalloids and Nonmetals
Compounds of Organometallic Elements

6. Science of Matter and Energy
Physics of Heat and Cold; Thermodynamics
The Kinetic Theory
Quantum Mechanics.
A Brief Introduction to Chemical Thermodynamics
Inorganic Chemistry

7. Chemical Analysis
Qualitative Methods
- Mathematical Dissection
Methods that Use Instruments
To analyse the spectrum
It's a Chromatograph

8. Biochemistry
Biology Molecules
In other words, enzymes
What Your Body Does All Day
Genes and RNA
Specific Proteins and Enzymes

9. Chemical Uses
Chemistry in Drug Production
Chemistry in the Environment
Science of Materials
Chemistry of Food
This is Nanotechnology.

10. What the Future Holds for Chemistry
Opportunities and Threats
Organic Synthesis
Cross-Disciplinary Study
Space Chemistry
Concerns of a Moral Nature

11. Conclusion
Summary of Vital Information
Constant Importance of Chemistry
Let's get started on our quest to learn everything we can about chemistry and discover why it's such an important and fascinating field of study.

1. Introduction

The Role of Chemistry in Everyday Life

The world we live in is shaped by chemistry, and it's everywhere. It's in the environment we live in, the water we consume, the food we eat, and the things we make and use. The behaviour of matter is fundamentally governed by chemistry, from the smallest molecule to the largest chemical reactions.

There are many reasons why this field of study is essential:

1. Chemistry aids our understanding of the structure and behaviour of the natural world. It clarifies the processes of photosynthesis in plants and the oxidation of metals.

2. Many recent technological advances can be traced back to the pioneering role played by chemistry. It has led to the development of life-saving pharmaceuticals, eco-friendly building materials, and cutting-edge energy saving gadgets.

3. Sustainable energy development, pollution reduction, and adaptation to a changing climate are just a few of the many environmental problems that chemistry can help solve.

4. In the medical field, chemistry plays a crucial role in the development of new drugs, diagnostic tools, and therapeutic procedures. It is crucial for medical researchers and practitioners to have a firm grasp on the chemistry of the human body.

5. Plastics, textiles, and electronics are just a few examples of products that rely on chemical processes throughout production. Industrial operations and product quality both stand to benefit from advances in chemistry.

6. Agriculture and Food: Chemistry has a role in all aspects of food creation, storage, and consumption. It aids in the creation of new food products and guarantees that they are up to par.

7. Chemistry plays an essential role in space exploration, from the development of rocket fuel and life support systems to the investigation of otherworldly landscapes.

8. Chemical processes underpin all forms of energy generation and storage, from fossil fuels and nuclear power to solar panels and rechargeable batteries.

Limits of the Topic at Hand

In this in-depth look of chemistry, we'll investigate everything from the field's early beginnings to its modern applications and potential in the future. The following sections make up our itinerary:

- A Brief History of Chemistry: We will explore the development of chemistry from its earliest days to the present day, focusing on seminal moments and seminal discoveries along the way.

- The Basics of Chemistry: In this section, we'll explore the building blocks of chemistry, from atoms and elements to chemical bonds and reactions.

Organic chemists investigate molecules with carbon atoms to learn more about their properties, applications, and reactions.

Metals, minerals, and nonmetals are all examples of molecules studied in inorganic chemistry since they do not predominantly consist of carbon-hydrogen (C-H) bonds.

Physical chemists investigate the fundamental laws that control chemical reactions and the material qualities of matter.

Analytical chemistry is the scientific study of separating substances into their component parts and determining precise amounts of those parts.

Biochemistry is the study of the chemical processes and chemicals that keep living things alive.

Applications of Chemistry: We'll look at chemistry's role in areas like medicine, materials research, environmental safeguards, and agriculture.

The emphasis on green chemistry, multidisciplinary study, and space travel are just a few of the topics that will be discussed in this chapter on the future of chemistry.

Finally, we will reflect on the continuing significance and relevance of chemistry in our lives by reviewing the main issues covered throughout this extensive investigation of the subject.

To kick off our adventure, let's learn more about the development of chemistry over the centuries.

2. An Outline of Chemical Development

When early humans first started to experiment with and learn about the characteristics of materials, this was the beginning of chemistry. The genesis of modern chemistry can be traced back to these early practises, which included metallurgy, dye manufacturing, and the brewing of alcoholic beverages.

The Way Back When

Alchemy, a metaphysical and philosophical tradition dating back thousands of years, is inextricably linked to the development of chemistry. The goal of alchemy, and the alchemists who pursued it, was to find a way to turn common metals like lead into more valuable ones like gold and to create an immortality-granting elixir.

Distillation, sublimation, and the employment of several tools and symbols were all common alchemical procedures. Although we

However, chemy's support of experimentation and the systematic study of matter was crucial in the development of modern chemistry.

Jabir ibn Hayyan, a Persian alchemist who flourished in the eighth century, is often regarded as one of the most important characters in the field's history. Many of the chemical procedures and laboratory methods developed in the centuries after Jabir's death owe their existence to his writings.

 The Evolution of Chemistry from Alchemy to the Present Day

It took several centuries, but alchemy eventually gave way to modern chemistry. This required a pivot away from alchemy's more esoteric spiritual roots and towards its more scientific examination of matter and its transmutations.

The rejection of the concept of the philosopher's stone, a mythological material that could turn base metals into gold and provide immortality, was a major turning point throughout this transition. Alchemists shifted their attention to fields where their expertise might be put to use, such as metalworking, glassmaking, and medicine.

Understanding of chemical processes made great strides in the 17th century. A more systematic approach of classifying matter was made possible by the concept of elements and compounds, which was introduced by Robert Boyle, commonly regarded one of the pioneers of modern chemistry. Boyle's research paved the way for the scientific method to be used to chemistry.

The Age of Chemical Progress

The term "Chemical Revolution" refers to the dramatic period of change in chemistry that occurred in the latter half of the 18th century. During this time period, Antoine Lavoisier, widely called the "Father of Modern Chemistry," emerged and revolutionised the profession with his discoveries about the conservation of mass and the discovery of chemical elements.

Through careful observation and experimentation, Lavoisier was able to formulate the rule of conservation of mass, which asserts that in chemical reactions, matter is neither generated nor destroyed but merely rearranges itself. The contemporary system of chemical nomenclature, which streamlined the naming of substances, was also largely due to his contributions.

Innovations of the 19th and 20th Centuries

Significant progress was made in chemistry during the 19th century. According to John Dalton's atomic hypothesis, all matter is made up of discrete particles called atoms. Understanding chemical reactions was made more rigorous by this hypothesis.

To forecast yet-to-be-discovered elements and establish the periodic rule, scientists used Dmitri Mendeleev's periodic chart, first published in 1869.

Chemistry made many more strides forward in the twentieth century. The advent of quantum mechanics led to a dramatic shift in our conceptualization of subatomic particles and their interactions. With this new information, scientists might make more precise predictions about chemical reactions and the properties of matter.

The scientific discipline of biochemistry, which investigates chemical processes within living beings, emerged in the middle of the 20th century. In 1953, James Watson and Francis Crick made a seminal discovery when they discovered the double helix structure of DNA.

Modern Chemical Processes

The modern field of chemistry is interdisciplinary and rapidly evolving. Nanotechnology, materials science, environmental chemistry, and many more are at the cutting edge of modern chemistry, and their study is expanding the field.

Climate change, pollution, and sustainable energy generation are just a few of the other major global issues that chemistry is helping to combat. The goal of green chemistry is to create chemical processes and materials that are less harmful to the environment.

Moving further, we shall investigate the underlying principles of chemistry to better understand this fascinating field.

3. Chemistry's Foundations

Elements and Atoms

The atomic theory is fundamental to the study of chemistry. The smallest unit of matter that can retain the chemical properties of its element is called an atom. Substances that contain only one sort of atom are called "elements." Chemical elements are classified in the periodic table according to their atomic number, which is the total number of protons in the nucleus.

There are three fundamental particles that make up an atom.

1. Atomic nuclei are composed of positively charged particles called protons. Atoms are classified according to their atomic number, which is based on the number of protons they contain.

2. The nucleus is home to neutral particles called neutrons. Neutrons add to the atom's mass but have no effect on its chemistry.

3. Electrons are subatomic particles with a negative charge that travel in shells around the nucleus. Bonding between atoms and chemical reactions both require electrons.

Synthetic Bonds

Atoms form molecules and compounds through a process called chemical bonding. When atoms join forces, they create a lower-energy, more stable structure. The three most common types of chemical bonding are as follows:

1. Cations and anions are two types of ions that are formed when one atom gives up an electron to another atom, creating a net positive and negative charge. Ionic compounds are formed when ions with opposite charges bind together. In the case of sodium chloride (table salt), the Na+ and Cl- ions form an ionic connection.

2. Covalent bonds are formed when electrons are shared between atoms in order to fill their outer electron shells. Molecules are formed when electrons are shared between atoms. Both polar (in which electrons are shared unequally) and nonpolar (in which electrons are shared equally) covalent bonds exist. In the H_2O molecule, for instance, the electrons of the oxygen (O) and hydrogen (H) atoms are shared.

3. Metallic bonding can be found in both metals and alloys. Metallic bonding allows electrons to travel freely around the metal's structure

without being localised. Metals' special features, like as electrical conductivity and malleability, can be traced back to their shared electron cloud.

Chemistry: The Reactions

In order to change reactants into products, chemical reactions require the breaking and formation of chemical bonds. According to the principle of mass conservation, in a chemical reaction, the sum of the masses of the reactants and the products must be equal. This law emphasises the concept that during chemical reactions, matter is conserved.

A chemical equation is a symbolic representation of a chemical process, giving a brief account of the reactants and products. One such instance is as follows:

$$2H_2 + O_2 \rightarrow 2H_2O$$

Hydrogen gas (H_2) and oxygen gas (O_2) combine to make water (H_2O) in this equation. The stoichiometry of a reaction is represented by the numbers in front of the chemical formulas (coefficients), which denote the ratio of reactants to products.

Periodic Table of Elements

Atomic number and electron configuration are used to create a tabular arrangement of the chemical elements known as the periodic table. It's helpful for learning about the physical and chemical characteristics of elements. Groups or families of components share comparable features and are displayed in the same column as their respective symbols.

There are a few main characteristics of the periodic table:

- The Periods in the periodic table are the horizontal columns. Periodically adjacent elements share a common number of electron shells.

Clusters: Rows of elements in the periodic table. The comparable chemical characteristics of elements can be attributed to their same valence electron count.

The group of elements in the centre of the periodic table called "transition metals" due to their range of oxidation states and metallic characteristics.

Group Noble Gases

There are 18 elements whose electron configurations are so stable that they cannot react chemically.

These elements, known as metalloids, share characteristics with both metals and nonmetals. Germanium (Ge) and silicon (Si) are two such elements.

For chemists, the periodic table is an indispensable resource for looking up information and making predictions about the properties and interactions of different elements.

Stoichiometry and Chemical Equations

The stoichiometry of a reaction can be represented in a chemical equation, which also serves as a simple representation of the reaction itself. The quantitative analysis of the components of a chemical process is called stoichiometry. Quantities like mass, moles, and volumes must be calculated, as well as the mole ratios of reactants and products.

Stoichiometry requires balancing chemical equations. By having the same amount of atoms of each element on both sides of the equation, a balanced equation guarantees that the law of conservation of mass is adhered to.

Let's look at a chemical equation for the formation of water from hydrogen and oxygen:

$$2H_2 + O_2 \rightarrow 2H_2O$$

Two molecules of hydrogen (H_2) and one molecule of oxygen (O_2) react to form two molecules of water (H_2O) in this balanced equation.

Calculations in stoichiometry include:

It is common practise to express the mass of a substance in terms of its molecular weight, or g/mol.

- Mole-to-Mole Conversions: converting between moles of reactants and moles of products using the coefficients in a balanced equation.

When converting between mass and moles, the molar mass of a substance is used.

The ideal gas law for gases is used to make the conversion from volume to moles.

Stoichiometry is an essential part of chemistry because it helps scientists calculate the exact amounts of materials used and those created during chemical reactions.

Now that we have a firm grasp of the cornerstones of chemistry, we can dive further into the specialised areas of study that make up the many subfields.

4. Molecular Biology

Natural Substances

The study of substances with carbon, or organic compounds, is the focus of organic chemistry. Although carbon is the most common element in organic molecules, other elements such as hydrogen, oxygen, nitrogen, and sulphur can also be present. Carbon's adaptability means it can be used to make compounds with a wide range of structures and properties.

Organic substances are ubiquitous in the natural world and absolutely necessary for survival. Synthetic substances like plastics, medicines, and pesticides are included, along with naturally occurring molecules including proteins, carbohydrates, lipids, and nucleic acids.

Hydrocarbons

Hydrocarbons are the simplest class of organic molecules, made up of just carbon and hydrogen. They are the building blocks of organic chemistry because they are the simplest type of organic molecules. There are two main classes of hydrocarbons, and these are:

1. Hydrocarbons that are referred to as "aliphatic" can have either unbranched or branched chains of carbon atoms. There are three more groups inside this larger one:
Saturated hydrocarbons consisting of only single bonds between carbon atoms are called "alkanes."
Alkenes are a class of unsaturated hydrocarbons that include at least one double bond.
Alkynes are a type of unsaturated hydrocarbon in which at least one of the carbon atom bonds is a triple bond.

2. Aromatic compounds have a benzene ring, which is a unique ring structure. These compounds are found in a wide variety of both natural and manmade substances, and their unusual features are a result of their resonance structures.

Groups With a Purpose

The distinctive chemical properties and reactivity of organic molecules are the result of the presence of functional groups, which are specific groupings of atoms within the molecules. In organic chemistry, functional groups are crucial because they determine the chemical reactions that can occur between organic molecules. These are examples of common functional groups:

Alcohol (-OH): The presence of the hydroxyl group gives alcohol desirable characteristics including water solubility and the ability to create hydrogen bonds.

Nucleophilic addition processes involve the carbonyl group, which is found in molecules like aldehydes and ketones.

Amines are nitrogen-containing organic molecules with a (-NH2) prefix. They can function as bases because nitrogen has an unshared pair of electrons.

Carboxylic acids have acidic qualities because the -OH group can transfer a proton (H+) to make them more basic.

Esters are used extensively in the flavour and fragrance business because to the pleasant, fruity aromas they produce.

Amides (-CONH2) are crucial to the structure and function of proteins and show a wide range of reactions in living organisms.

Isomorphism

When two or more compounds share the same chemical formula but have distinct structural arrangements or spatial orientations, this is called isomerism in organic chemistry. Despite sharing the same atoms and the same number of each atom type, isomers can display varying chemical characteristics and reactivity.

Isomerism can be broken down into two categories:

Structural isomers differ in how their atoms are arranged, hence the name. This comprises functional group isomerism, position isomerism, and chain isomerism, all of which refer to variations in the arrangement of functional groups within a molecule.

- Stereoisomerism: Stereoisomers share the same molecular formula but have a different atomic or group spatial orientation. Geometric (cis-trans) isomerism and optical (enantiomeric) isomerism fall under this category.

Isomerism increases the difficulty of studying organic compounds and highlights the value of learning about molecules in three dimensions.

Mechanisms of Reactions,

Every chemical reaction in organic chemistry has its own unique mechanism and reaction pathway. The chemical details of how molecules of reactants are converted into molecules of products are described in reaction mechanisms. It is essential to comprehend these mechanisms in order to foretell the results of organic reactions.

Here are some examples of frequent organic reactions and the corresponding mechanisms:

Substitution reactions are chemical processes in which one molecular group is exchanged for another. Nucleophilic substitution and electrophilic substitution are two processes that can bring this about.

Reactions in which atoms or groups are added to an existing molecule are called "addition reactions." Alkene and alkyne addition reactions are one such example.

The elimination of an atom or group from a molecule is the end result of elimination processes. E1 and E2 reactions are frequent instances of this type.

Gaining an electron occurs during reduction, while losing an electron occurs during oxidation. Inorganic chemistry relies heavily on redox reactions.

Pharmaceuticals, petrochemicals, polymers, and even agriculture all rely heavily on the findings of organic chemists. It paves the way for the synthesis and manipulation of organic molecules for uses ranging from medication design to sustainable material production.

5. Organic Chemistry

Inorganic Substances

Compounds that do not predominately consist of carbon-hydrogen (C-H) bonds are the primary focus of inorganic chemistry. Metals, minerals, salts, and coordination compounds are all part of inorganic chemistry, which covers a much broader range of substances than organic chemistry, which focuses on carbon-containing compounds.

There is a wide range of uses for inorganic chemicals. Some Prominent

Table salt (sodium chloride), rust (iron oxide), and quartz (silicon dioxide) are all examples of inorganic compounds. The study of minerals and rocks, as well as the production of metals, rely heavily on the principles of inorganic chemistry.

Combinatorial Chemistry

Complex compounds, or coordination compounds, are widely studied in the field of inorganic chemistry. A metal atom or ion is at the centre of these compounds, and it is surrounded by other molecules or ions that serve as ligands. In order to donate electrons to the metal centre, ligands tend to be electron-rich species containing lone pairs of electrons.

The number of ligand molecules or ions covalently bound to a metal in a complex is referred to as the coordination number of that metal. Catalysis, bioinorganic chemistry, and materials science all rely heavily on the diverse set of capabilities and colours displayed by coordination compounds.

Elements in Transition

The transition metals are a colourful collection of elements that can be found in the middle of the periodic table and have a wide range of oxidation states. They are essential in a wide variety of industrial and biological processes.

The following are examples of popular uses for transition metals:

Haemoglobin, which carries oxygen in the blood, and the iron needed to make steel and other alloys are both made of this element.

Copper (Cu) is a metal that has several practical applications, including in plumbing, electrical wiring, and as a catalyst in chemistry.

Cobalt (Co) is a component of vitamin B12 and is used in the manufacturing of powerful magnets.

You can get chromium (Cr) in stainless steel and corrosion-resistant finishes.

Nickel (Ni) is a metal used to make steel and other alloys.

Manganese (Mn): Required for photosynthesis in plants; also found in steel and battery manufacture.

Inorganic compounds and metalloids

Nonmetals and metalloids, which are elements with characteristics in between those of metals and nonmetals, are also studied in inorganic chemistry.

To the right of the metals on the periodic table are the nonmetals, which include hydrogen, oxygen, nitrogen, and sulphur. Different molecular forms of these materials exist, but in general they are poor heat and electrical conductors.

Some elements, known as "metalloids," have characteristics typical of both metals and nonmetals. Si, Ge, and As are all elements that fit this description. Semiconductor technology relies heavily on metalloids.

From the minerals that make up the Earth's crust to the complex coordination compounds utilised in medicine and industry, inorganic chemistry is a broad area that investigates the characteristics, structures, and reactivity of many different substances.

6. Chemistry, Physical

In the realm of thermodynamics,

Thermodynamics is the study of energy and its transformations in chemical systems, and it is a subfield of physical chemistry. It sheds light on the impromptu nature of chemical reactions and the pathways they take. The fundamental ideas of thermodynamics are:

Energy can be broken down into two categories: kinetic (energy of motion) and potential (energy that has been stored). Heat (q) and work (w) are common forms of energy transformation in chemical systems.

Energy cannot be created or destroyed in a closed system, as stated by the First rule of Thermodynamics, sometimes known as the "law of conservation of energy." All it can do is shapeshift. Internal energy change (U) is defined mathematically as the difference between heat input (q) and work output (w).

The degree of disorder in a system is represented by a number called entropy (S), which is the subject of the Second Law of Thermodynamics. According to the second rule of thermodynamics, entropy always tends to grow over time because the potential energy of a state is always smaller than that of its starting state if no energy enters or exits the system.

The Gibbs free energy (G) is a thermodynamic potential that incorporates both enthalpy (H) and entropy (S) to make predictions about the spontaneity of a reaction. A negative value for G indicates a spontaneous reaction; a positive value indicates a nonspontaneous reaction; and a value of zero indicates that the system is in equilibrium.

- Enthalpy and Entropy: Enthalpy (H) is the overall heat content of a system, while entropy (S) is the degree of disorder or unpredictability in that system. The degree to which a reaction occurs spontaneously depends on the change in enthalpy (H) and entropy (S).

The Kinetics of Everything

Chemical kinetics is the study of reaction rates and the variables that affect them. It digs into how reactions work and the aspects that can be adjusted to regulate reaction times. The fundamental ideas of kinetics are:

The rate of a reaction is defined as the rate at which the concentration of reactants or products changes for a given amount of time. Moles per litre per second is a common unit of measurement.

The rate law describes the link between the concentrations of reactants and the rate of the reaction. It is experimentally determined and may be different for various reactions.

- Reaction Mechanism: This term refers to the breakdown of a more involved reaction into its component parts. Short-lived species that form during a chemical reaction are included in this category, as are intermediates and reaction intermediates.

- Activation Energy (Ea) is the minimum energy input required to initiate a reaction. It is the amount of energy needed to convert one mole of a reactant into one mole of a product.

Catalysis is the process by which the pace of a chemical reaction is increased without the catalyst itself being used up. They do this by making the response less energetically demanding to start.

- Collision Theory: According to this theory, molecules of the reactants must collide with enough energy and in the right orientation for a reaction to take place. Only collisions with sufficient energy (more than the activation energy) result in a reaction.

Predicting the behaviour of chemical reactions in different conditions, optimising industrial chemical processes, and creating effective catalytic devices all require an understanding of reaction kinetics.

Quantum mechanics,

The field of physical chemistry known as quantum mechanics investigates the fundamental interactions between matter and energy at the subatomic level. It offers a theoretical basis for deducing the inner workings of atoms and molecules' electronic structures. The following are important ideas in quantum mechanics:

- Wave-Particle Duality: According to quantum mechanics, elementary particles like electrons can behave in two different ways: as waves and as particles. This duality is crucial to grasping the nature of quantum particle behaviour.

The probability density of an electron's location around an atom is described by wave functions. They are used to calculate electron configurations and have a mathematical representation.

Quantum mechanics states that the energy levels of atoms and molecules are quantized, or limited to a small range of values. The idea of energy levels and electron shells follows from this.

The Schrödinger Equation is the backbone of quantum mechanics. It is used to describe how electrons behave within an atom or molecule and to compute attributes like energy levels and electron distributions.

According to the Orbital Theory, electrons can be found in certain locations in space called orbitals. Specific quantum numbers, such as the primary quantum number (n), angular momentum quantum number (l), and magnetic quantum number (m), are used to identify them.

1.2 Historical Overview of Chemistry

Chemistry: A Brief History

The history of chemistry as a scientific field spans aeons and is replete with breakthroughs and paradigm shifts. The history of chemistry is a tribute to human inquisitiveness and the unrelenting desire of understanding the natural world, from its origins in the mystical practises of alchemy to its contemporary place as a core science. In this survey, we will follow the development of chemistry and emphasise significant turning points and the work of influential individuals.

The Way Back When

Chemistry has its roots in the early civilizations' use of materials and the resulting understanding of their properties. These traditional methods were crucial to the growth of contemporary chemistry.

Mesopotamia and Egypt's Rich Past

Metal extraction and alloy production were both pioneered in ancient Egypt and Mesopotamia approximately 4000 BCE. They also produced ceramics, glassware, and metalwork at an early stage. To accomplish this, one needed knowledge of the characteristics and transformation mechanisms of various chemicals.

China's Classical Era

The ancient Chinese chemical community made important discoveries. Distilling alcohol and making gunpowder were only two of the many chemical processes that Chinese alchemists experimented on as early as the fifth century BCE. The foundation for future chemical progress was laid by these discoveries.

Greek Antiquity

Empedocles and Democritus, two ancient Greek philosophers, put forth pioneering theories about the make-up of matter. Empedocles postulated that all matter is composed of the same four elements: earth, water, air, and fire. Democritus, on the other hand, suggested that matter was made up of indivisible particles he named "atomos," establishing the framework for the atomic theory.

The Evolution of Chemistry from Alchemy to the Present Day

Over the course of several centuries, chemistry evolved from the mystical and spiritual practises of alchemy to the more systematic and scientific approach of contemporary chemistry.

A Golden Era in Islamic History

The Islamic Golden Age extended from the eighth to the thirteenth centuries, and it was during this time that Islamic academics achieved great advances in the field of alchemy. Jabir ibn Hayyan, better known in the West as Geber, was an important player in the development of alchemy. The systematic investigation of matter and the employment of experimental methods and equipment were major themes in Jabir's writings.

The Rhazes of Al-Razi

In the 9th century, the Persian genius Al-Razi revolutionised chemistry with his discoveries. Distillation and crystallisation are just two of the many chemical processes that he is credited with developing. The methodical approach to chemistry that Al-Razi introduced paved the way for later developments.

The Age of Enlightenment in Europe

During the European Renaissance, alchemy and the quest for knowledge gained fresh popularity. European alchemists looked for a way to turn common metals into gold and for the fabled philosopher's stone, which they thought would grant immortality. Despite being motivated by esoteric concerns, these investigations paved the way for modern laboratory practises and the systematic study of matter.

The Age of Chemical Progress

The field of chemistry underwent a radical change, known as the Chemical Revolution, in the latter half of the 18th century. During this time, the world met Antoine Lavoisier, widely regarded as the "Father of Modern Chemistry."

Lavoisier, Antoine,

Antoine Lavoisier's research paved the way for modern chemistry and fundamentally altered our knowledge of chemical interactions. The law of conservation of mass, which asserts that in chemical reactions, matter is not generated nor destroyed but just rearranged, was formulated based on his careful investigations. Lavoisier's research was crucial in debunking the then-outdated phlogiston theory, which had been developed to explain combustion.

Lavoisier also pioneered the idea of chemical elements and compounds, which allowed for the first systematic approach to arranging different forms of matter. The contemporary system of chemical nomenclature, which greatly reduced the complexity of identifying substances, was established in large part due to his efforts.

Innovations of the 19th and 20th Centuries

Significant progress in the knowledge of chemical principles and the development of modern chemistry occurred in the 19th and 20th century.

John Dalton

The concept of atoms as the fundamental building blocks of matter was first postulated by John Dalton in the early 19th century in his atomic theory. Dalton postulated that atoms of different masses make up each element, and that atomic rearrangement lies at the heart of chemical reactions. Dalton's contributions established a more solid groundwork for our knowledge of chemical processes.

Dmitri Mendeleev

To organise the known elements according to their properties and atomic weights, Dmitri Mendeleev released his periodic table in 1869. Mendeleev was able to forecast the presence and qualities of elements that had not yet been discovered thanks to his periodic table, which did more than just group elements with similar properties together. The periodic table is still indispensable to chemists today.

This is Quantum Mechanics,

Understanding how matter behaves at the atomic and subatomic levels underwent a revolutionary shift in the 20th century. In order to comprehend how the electrons in an atom or molecule are arranged, physicists like Max Planck, Albert Einstein, Niels Bohr, and Erwin Schrödinger created the theory known as quantum mechanics.

Particles like electrons, according to the wave-particle duality postulated by quantum physics, can act in both wave and particle modes. This theory enabled for accurate estimates of energy levels and electron distributions, completely transforming our knowledge of atomic and molecule interactions.

Chemistry of Life

Biochemistry as a distinct scientific discipline also emerged in the twentieth century. Studying biomolecules including proteins, nucleic acids, lipids, and carbohydrates, biochemists investigate the chemical processes that sustain life. In 1953, James Watson and Francis Crick made a groundbreaking discovery when they determined the structure of DNA.

Modern Chemical Processes

The modern field of chemistry is interdisciplinary and rapidly evolving. Organic chemistry, inorganic chemistry, physical chemistry, analytical chemistry, and biochemistry are just some of the many subfields that fall under the umbrella of chemistry.

Eco-Friendly Synthesis

The creation of environmentally friendly chemical processes is one of the most pressing problems facing the chemical industry today. The goal of "green chemistry" is to develop chemical processes and products that are harmless to both the environment and human health while still being profitable. Its goals include cutting down on harmful pollutants, recycling more, and using renewable energy.

Research That Bridges Disciplines

Interdisciplinary study is on the rise as a result of chemistry's growing interdisciplinarity. Research in materials science, for instance, focuses on tailoring the properties of novel materials for use in industries like electronics, aircraft, and healthcare.

Nanotechnology is an interdisciplinary study of how to control matter at the nanoscale to make novel materials and gadgets.

The Chemistry of Outer Space

Space travel and the study of otherworldly settings rely heavily on the field of chemistry. Scientists use analytical and inorganic chemistry methods to determine the chemical make-up of extraterrestrial objects like planets, moons, and comets. To successfully explore other planets and look for life beyond Earth, astronauts need a firm grasp of the chemistry of space.

Concerns From An Ethical Standpoint

As the field of chemistry develops, the importance of moral questions has grown. The ethical use of chemicals, the creation of rules for doing research in an ethical manner, and the effects of chemical technology on human society and the natural environment are all issues that chemists must consider.

Summary

The

A look back at the development of chemistry across time shows a fascinating tale of scientific discovery and discovery itself. The field of chemistry has developed and broadened over time, from the early practises of alchemy to the methodical and rigorous science of today. In addition to expanding our knowledge of the natural world, the discoveries and improvements made possible by chemists have had a profound impact on the development of technology and the way we live today. Chemistry's continued development places it at the front of efforts to solve global problems and expand the boundaries of our understanding of the natural world.

Chapter 2:
The Structure of Atoms

2.1 The Atom: Building Block of Matter

Sub-Material Unit, or Atom

The atom is one of the most fundamental notions in all of science. This minuscule, cryptic particle is the stuff of which everything is made and the bedrock upon which the cosmos rests. The history of the atom is a tribute to the strength of human curiosity and inventiveness, and it spans millennia of exploration, experimentation, and discovery.

Democritus and Leucippus, two ancient Greek philosophers, believed that all matter is made up of fundamental, unbreakable particles they named "atomos," from the Greek for "uncuttable" or "indivisible." Although mostly hypothetical and lacking empirical support, this early theory established the framework for our present understanding of the atom.

Not until the turn of the nineteenth century did the idea of the atom start to take shape. In 1803, English chemist John Dalton proposed his atomic hypothesis, which held that all matter is made up of extremely small, unbreakable units called atoms. Dalton's hypothesis was an important step forward in our knowledge of the atom since it gave a framework for analysing chemical reactions and the behaviour of gases.

That various elements' atoms have varying weights and mix in fixed ratios to produce compounds was a major discovery of Dalton's atomic theory. The idea behind it led to the creation of the periodic table, which is still used as a standard reference in chemistry today.

Scientists began to delve more deeply into the atomic structure as the 19th century advanced. The electron, a negatively charged particle, was first recognised as a component of atoms by J.J. Thomson in 1897. First experimental evidence that atoms have a substructure was found thanks to Thomson's efforts.

In Thomson's 'plum pudding' model of the atom, the positively charged 'pudding' of matter is said to surround the electrons. This model was a big change from Dalton's indivisible atoms, but it still didn't explain all about the atom's interior.

In 1909, Ernest Rutherford made the next crucial discovery towards atomic comprehension. The famous gold foil experiment was performed by Rutherford, in which alpha particles (positively charged particles) were fired at a thin sheet of gold foil. Some of the alpha particles were deflected at sharp angles, which he interpreted to mean that the atom contained a small, compact, positively charged nucleus.

The atomic structure is now better understood thanks to Rutherford's discovery. It showed that the nucleus of an atom contains positively charged protons and that the atom itself is not a homogeneous pudding. The negatively charged electrons lingered in distant orbit around the nucleus.

The Danish physicist Niels Bohr further developed the atomic idea with his Bohr model in 1913. It was Bohr's contention that electrons circulated in predetermined energy levels or orbits around the nucleus. This model not only lay the framework for our current understanding of atomic and molecular behaviour, but it also provided a successful explanation for the spectral lines of hydrogen.

In the early 20th century, atomic physics made tremendous strides forward. The Schrödinger equation, developed by Erwin Schrödinger in 1926, is a mathematical description of the motion of electrons within atoms. Due to the incorporation of the wave-particle duality of electrons and the probabilistic nature of their behaviour, this quantum mechanical model provides a more precise and full account of atomic structure.

The uncertainty principle, proposed by Werner Heisenberg in tandem with Schrödinger's work, states that it is impossible to know with absolute certainty the position and momentum of a particle at the same time. This principle emphasised the probabilistic aspect of quantum mechanics and radically altered our perception of the subatomic world.

Further discoveries and breakthroughs in atomic physics were made during the middle of the twentieth century. Neutrons are electrically neutral particles that can be found in the nucleus of atoms, and their existence was verified by James Chadwick in 1932. This finding rounded up our understanding of the atomic structure by adding neutrons to the previously identified protons and electrons.
The development of nuclear physics allowed for a fuller investigation of the atomic nucleus and its properties. In the 1930s and 1940s, scientists were able to analyse the properties of atomic nuclei and discover the forces that kept them together thanks to the advent of nuclear reactors and particle accelerators.

The discovery of nuclear fission by Otto Hahn and Fritz Strassmann in 1938 was a major advance in the field of nuclear physics. This discovery paved the way for the creation of nuclear weapons and nuclear power by showing that when an atomic nucleus divides into two smaller nuclei, a great quantity of energy is released.

The Manhattan Project's creation of the atomic bomb during World War II changed the world and ushered in the nuclear era. The atomic bomb's devastating effects have refocused attention on the importance of making safe, ethical use of nuclear science and technology.Particle accelerators and the study of subatomic particles both contributed to the further advancement of atomic physics after World War II. New particles, including as mesons and neutrinos, have added to our knowledge of the underlying components and forces that shape the cosmos.

The Standard Model of particle physics, developed in the latter half of the 20th century, is the most robust theoretical framework for describing the fundamental particles and their interactions. This model successfully explained a wide variety of experimental data since it encompassed the electromagnetic, weak, and strong nuclear forces.

Our knowledge of the atom is more refined now than it has ever been. We know that atoms have a nucleus made of protons and neutrons and that the nucleus is surrounded by a cloud of electrons with different energy levels. From the electromagnetic force that keeps electrons in their orbits to the strong nuclear force that keeps protons and neutrons bound together in the nucleus, we have a firm grasp on the many forces that govern the actions of subatomic particles.

We have also uncovered a plethora of subatomic particles including quarks, neutrinos, and bosons that are essential to the basic interactions in the cosmos. Particle physics research has improved our understanding of the universe at all scales, from the subatomic to the galactic.

The atom has not only played a crucial role in physics, but also in chemistry and technology. Materials science, health, and electronics stand to benefit greatly from nanotechnology, which emerged as a result of atomic-scale atom and molecule manipulation.

The periodic table was developed to categorise chemical elements according to their atomic number and properties, thanks to our increased knowledge of atomic structure. Chemists rely heavily on this table to make predictions about the properties of elements and compounds and to create new materials with tailored characteristics.

The atom is also essential in the generation of energy. A relatively clean and efficient energy source, nuclear power plants convert the energy released during nuclear fission into electricity. Nuclear power has the potential to greatly benefit society, but it also brings up serious concerns about safety, waste management, and the spread of nuclear weapons.

The history of the atom is a powerful illustration of how human curiosity and the pursuit of knowledge may change the world. Our quest to understand the atom has been astounding, spanning from the theoretical thoughts of the ancient Greeks to the present day understanding of quantum physics and the Standard Model.

Science is a dynamic endeavour, and our knowledge of the cosmos is constantly being updated and improved as a result.

As the fundamental unit of matter, the atom is crucial to our efforts to understand the universe and harness its power for the benefit of humanity.

We have to consider the moral and societal repercussions of our findings as we push the envelope of atomic physics and expand our understanding. The atom's potential as both an energy source and a weapon of mass destruction highlights the importance of maintaining scientific integrity.

In conclusion, the atom is the basic building block of matter, and the study of it has profoundly influenced human development. The history of the atom, from the first theories of ancient philosophers to the cutting-edge concepts of modern quantum physics, is a monument to human curiosity, inventiveness, and the transformative power of scientific inquiry. The more we learn about the atomic world, the more we have a responsibility to use that information for the benefit of all people and the preservation of our home planet. One of the deepest and longest-lasting topics of scientific inquiry, the atom retains all its complexity and relevance to this day.

2.2 Subatomic Particles: Protons, Neutrons, Electrons

The Proton, Neutron, and Electron Are All Subatomic Particles

The tale of matter is woven into the intricate fabric of the universe at a scale so small that it strains our ability to comprehend it. The fundamental components of matter, known as subatomic particles, are located deep within this microscopic world. The building blocks of the universe are the subatomic particles known as protons, neutrons, and electrons. The story of these atomic heroes is an exploration of the depths of particle physics, a narrative that displays the sophistication and intricacy of the building blocks of our universe.

All matter is made up of atoms, which are made up of protons, neutrons, and electrons. The 20th century saw the discovery and explication of these particles, which greatly influenced our view of the physical world.

Neutral atoms that have positive protons.

The nucleus of an atom is filled with positively charged subatomic particles called protons. Ernest Rutherford discovered them in his now-famous gold foil experiment in 1909. Rutherford's seminal experiment demonstrated the existence of a small, dense nucleus at the atom's centre, where the vast majority of the atom's mass and positive charge are concentrated. There are protons in this nucleus.

The positive charge of a proton is the same size as the negative charge of an electron, but in the opposite direction. The electrical interactions that govern the behaviour of matter have their origins in this basic feature. The proton is a vital part of the element identification process. The position of an element on the periodic table is determined by its atomic number, which is equal to the number of protons in the nucleus of that element. Carbon atoms have exactly six protons, and oxygen atoms have exactly eight protons.

Even though protons are required to determine an element's identity, there are still many unknowns about them. There are two "up" quarks and one "down" quark in each of these tinier particles. These quarks are held together in the proton by the strong nuclear force, which is mediated by gluons. This internal organisation further increases the intricate nature of the subatomic realm.

The Neutral Stabilisers, or Neutrons

Like protons, neutrons are found in an atom's nucleus. However, they are distinct in one critical respect: they are not electrically charged. The discovery of neutrons by James Chadwick in 1932 rounded out our understanding of the atomic nucleus and solidified the neutron's place in the subatomic ensemble.

Neutrons are the "glue" that keeps the positively charged protons in the nucleus from scattering. Without neutrons, the nucleus would disintegrate due to electrostatic repulsion between protons. Because of this stabilising effect, atoms and, by extension, all matter in the universe are possible.

Like protons, neutrons have a multipart structure. Three quarks make them up, and the strong nuclear force is what keeps them together. Atomic nuclei are stable when attractive strong nuclear force is in equilibrium with repulsive electrostatic force between protons and neutrons within the nucleus. Because of this nuanced dynamic, nature contains a wide range of elemental and isotopic compositions.

Electrons are the orbits with a negative charge.
Negatively charged electrons travel in a circular path around the nucleus of an atom. In the early 20th century, scientists like J.J.

Thomson laid the groundwork for proving their existence. Compared to protons and neutrons, electrons have the smallest mass and are therefore the least massive of the three fundamental particles.

The chemical characteristics and behaviour of an atom are largely determined by its electrons. They are structured around the nucleus into shells of increasing energy. As electrons move from the innermost to the outermost shell, each energy level is filled to capacity.

Quantum mechanics, the field of physics that describes the behaviour of particles on the lowest sizes, governs the actions of electrons within an atom. Quantum mechanics states that electrons do not move in regular patterns like planets do when they orbit the sun. Instead, they are found in "electron clouds," which are essentially probability distributions for where an electron might be. It is axiomatic in quantum physics that the behaviour of electrons is probabilistic.

Chemical processes, enabled by electrons, form the basis for the wide variety of molecules and materials found in nature. Electrons in the outermost shells of atoms are the ones that interact with one another when they bond to form molecules. Sharing, transfer, or pooling of electrons between atoms results in chemical bonds, including covalent, ionic, and metallic connections.

It is essential for chemists and materials scientists to have a firm grasp on how electrons are distributed within atoms. The elements' properties may be predicted and understood in a systematic manner thanks to the periodic table, which is organised by atomic number.

Electrons have a crucial part in the operation of electronic equipment, in addition to their involvement in chemistry. Common electricity is the result of electrons moving across conductors. Electrons are not only the carriers of charge but also the backbone of modern technology because they are used to power everything from light bulbs to computers.

The Interplay of Forces Between Subatomic Particles

Gravity, electromagnetism, the strong nuclear force, and the weak nuclear force are the four fundamental forces that regulate the actions of subatomic particles. Each of these forces has a unique impact on the atomic level and beyond.

The force that controls the motion of huge objects on cosmic scales is called "Gravity." Despite being the weakest of the four basic forces, gravity causes all objects with mass to interact attractively with one another. However, at the atomic and subatomic scales, its impacts are often insignificant.

- Electromagnetism: Electromagnetism includes electric and magnetic interactions as a single fundamental force. It's what makes like charges repel one another and opposite charges (like electrons and protons) attract one another electromagnetically. Light and other electromagnetic waves are governed by the same principles of electromagnetism.

The strong nuclear force is the most potent of the four known basic interactions. It's what holds atomic nuclei together, holding protons and neutrons in place. The stability of atomic nuclei can be attributed to the strong nuclear force, which is mediated by particles called gluons.

When a neutron undergoes beta decay, for example, it splits into a proton, an electron, and an antineutrino as a result of the weak nuclear force. The weak nuclear force is important in the processes that power the sun and other stars, although being weaker than the other forces.

Learning how these forces interact is crucial to deciphering the nature of stuff and the cosmos. Atoms, the fundamental constituents of matter, join together through the interplay of these forces to form molecules, compounds, and the myriad other substances that make up our world.

The Quest for Unity in Particle Physics: Beyond the Atom

The most common atoms are protons, neutrons, and electrons, but there is a much more diverse and intricate universe at the subatomic level. The study of subatomic particles, known as "particle physics," has revealed a vast zoo of subatomic particles, each with its own distinct properties and behaviours.

Protons and neutrons, for instance, are composed of fundamental particles called quarks. There are six different "fl

particles called hadrons, and are never seen on their own.

The electron and neutrino both belong to a class of fundamental particles called leptons. Neutrinos are extremely difficult to catch because they are neutral electrically and have very weak interactions with materials. They are created in a number of different astronomical phenomena, including solar nuclear fusion and supernova explosions.

Bosons, on the other hand, are particles that convey forces and act as mediators of nature's fundamental interactions. For instance, the photon mediates the electromagnetic force, and the gluon transports the strong nuclear force, both of which are bosons. The Higgs boson is responsible for giving other particles their mass, and the W and Z bosons mediate the weak nuclear force.

The Standard Model is an all-encompassing theoretical framework that describes the electromagnetic, weak, and strong nuclear forces and accounts for the behaviour of most known subatomic particles, and it was developed as part of the quest for unity in particle physics. The Standard Model has been quite useful in understanding many different kinds of occurrences, although it does have some restrictions.

Reconciling the Standard Model with gravity as defined by Einstein's general theory of relativity is one of the most difficult problems in contemporary particle physics. Due to the failure of previous attempts to reconcile gravity with the other fundamental forces, the search for a theory of quantum gravity continues.

In addition, the majority of the mass and energy in the universe are made up of dark matter and dark energy, which are not accounted for by the Standard Model. These mysterious cosmological features continue to be a major unsolved mystery in contemporary astrophysics and cosmology.

The Universe and the Nature of Subatomic Particles

The history of the nucleons (protons, neutrons, and electrons) does not stay in the lab or in the theoretical physics world. It permeates the entire universe and determines the course of time and space.

Protons, neutrons, and electrons formed from the primordial soup of high-energy particles in the early universe. Hydrogen and helium were the first atoms to create as the universe cooled and expanded. Under the pull of gravity, these atoms began to coalesce, eventually forming the stars, galaxies, and other features of the modern cosmos.

Our sun and other stars like it are immense nuclear furnaces where protons fuse hydrogen into helium and release tremendous amounts of energy. The heavier elements like carbon, oxygen, and iron are created through nuclear fusion, which is powered by this energy and provided by the stars.

These newly produced elements are dispersed throughout the cosmos by the cataclysmic supernova explosions that occur when large stars run out of nuclear fuel. These debris become the raw material for new stars and planets, including our own home planet Earth.

Subatomic particle behaviour persists in moulding Earth's geology, climate, and biology. An internal heat source that affects the dynamics of Earth's core and mantle is radioactive decay, which is driven by the weak nuclear force. Plate tectonics, volcanic eruptions, and the uplift of mountain ranges are all results of this heat.

Electron behaviour in molecules is crucial to understanding the chemistry of life. Sharing and transferring electrons between atoms and molecules drives the metabolic processes that keep live creatures going.

Conclusion

The history of the proton, neutron, and electron is illustrative of human ingenuity and the efficacy of scientific investigation. Over the course of a century, scientists have discovered and analysed these subatomic particles, revealing insights into the nature of matter and energy on scales ranging from the subatomic to the cosmic.

The history of these elementary particles demonstrates the incredible interdependence of all things. The actions of protons, neutrons, and electrons echo throughout the cosmos, creating the physical and chemical processes that drive the variety and complexity of our universe, from the birth of galaxies and stars to the chemistry of life on Earth.

New mysteries and questions arise as our knowledge of the subatomic realm expands, encouraging us to push the boundaries of particle physics even farther. Unification, the hunt for dark matter and dark energy, and the investigation of nature's fundamental forces are all continuing to motivate scientific inquiry and test the limits of our understanding of the cosmos.

The history of the three fundamental particles (proton, neutron, and electron) is more than a scientific tale; it is a metaphor for humanity's search for meaning in the cosmos. These essential constituents of matter encourage us to probe the nature of reality, investigate the cosmos at its most elemental level, and marvel at the wonders of nature in all its forms.

Chapter 3:
Periodic Table

3.1 Organization of the Periodic Table

Schematic Presentation of the Elements

The periodic table of elements is a classic and indispensable resource for chemists everywhere. The elements, the building blocks of all matter in the cosmos, are graphically represented here. In order to study these elements and learn about their properties, interactions, and behaviours, scientists use the periodic table. We will examine the development, structure, and useful information that the periodic table provides for scientists and students alike.

Development in the Past

It took decades of teamwork, creativity, and discovery to get at today's periodic table. Antoine Lavoisier, in the late 18th century, was the first to classify chemical elements according to their characteristics. However, the first widely accepted periodic chart dates back to 1869 and was created by Russian chemist Dmitri Mendeleev.

The true genius of Mendeleev was his ability to predict the appearance of previously unknown elements. After sorting the elements by their atomic mass, he found that those with comparable qualities tended to appear in clusters at regular intervals. Mendeleev hypothesised the properties of unaccounted-for elements to preserve this order and fill in the gaps in his table. When these elements were eventually identified, their properties remarkably matched his predictions, lending credence to his periodic table.

As our knowledge of atomic structure grew, so did the periodic table. British scientist Henry Moseley made a seminal contribution in the early 20th century when he proposed using an element's atomic number—the total number of protons in its nucleus—to classify it. This modification resulted in the current version of the periodic table, which is more in line with the fundamental properties of atoms.

Periodic Table Organisation.

The elements of the periodic table are laid out in a grid with their own symbols and identifying data such as atomic number, mass, and chemical symbol. Elements' behaviour can be better understood and predicted thanks to the insights provided by its structure.

The rows of the table are designated as "periods," while the columns are labelled "groups." Because they all contain the same amount of valence electrons (the electrons in the outermost energy level of an atom), elements in the same group tend to exhibit comparable characteristics and chemical behaviours.

The rows of the periodic table are referred to as "periods." A higher electron energy level, or "shell," corresponds to each cycle. The addition of protons and electrons is represented by an increase in the atomic number as you read over a period from left to right. As you get to the right of the periodic table, you move away from the metals, which are on the left.

Groups, or families, are what the periodic table's vertical columns are referred to as. Because they share the same amount of valence electrons, elements in the same group tend to have comparable chemical characteristics. The current periodic table divides elements into 18 distinct groups, each of which is identified by a number and sometimes a letter.

The periodic table is broken down even further into distinct zones, each with its own set of characteristics:

Group 1 elements, such as lithium (Li), sodium (Na), and potassium (K), easily combine with other elements to produce compounds.

Group 2 elements like magnesium (Mg) and calcium (Ca) are metals like the alkali metals but are less reactive.

Well-known metals like iron (Fe), copper (Cu), and gold (Au) are examples of Transition Metals, which inhabit groups 3 to 12. The compounds of transition metals tend to be brightly coloured and easily shaped.

Halogens (Fluorine, Chlorine, and Iodine) are members of Group 17 and are highly reactive nonmetals that rapidly form salts when mixed with metals.

5. Noble Gases: Elements in Group 18 that are inert and non-radioactive, such as helium (He), neon (Ne), and argon (Ar). There is no smell or colour to these gases.

Carbon (C), nitrogen (N), and oxygen (O) are examples of nonmetals that can be found on the right side of the periodic table. They range from solid to liquid to gas in their physical state.

Metalloids, found in the zigzag region of the periodic table, are elements that have characteristics with both metals and nonmetals. Silicon (Si) and germanium (Ge) are two well-known examples of metalloids.

The eighth row of the periodic table consists of the Lanthanides and the Actinides, which are often located below the main body of the chart. Among these uses is the creation of powerful permanent magnets, which requires the usage of lanthanides. Heavy radioactive elements like uranium (U) and thorium (Th) are classified as actinides.

Tendencies and Structures

The structure of the periodic table provides scientists with a framework for identifying patterns and relationships among the elements. These tendencies guide scientific inquiry and practical applications by illuminating the nature and behaviour of components. Some of the more notable tendencies are:

One, Atomic Size: Across periods, atomic size falls, whereas within groups, it grows from top to bottom. The growth in nucleon size and the accumulation of electron shells are the primary causes of this pattern.

The energy needed to rip one electron out of an atom is called its "ionisation energy." Within a set, it tends to rise from bottom to top and fall from left to right as time progresses. In general, cations (ions with a positive charge) are more easily formed from elements with a lower ionisation energy.

The third property is an element's Electronegativity, which is its propensity to attract electrons in a chemical bond. From one time period to the next, it rises, and from one group to the next, it falls. In general, elements with a higher electronegativity are more likely to break down into anions (negatively charged ions).

To what extent an element displays metallike characteristics like malleability, ductility, and conductivity is defined by its metallic character. Across time, it rises from right to left, and inside a set, it rises from highest to lowest. The most metallic elements are found in the periodic table's bottom left corner.

5. Chemical Reactivity: Elements in the same group share the same amount of valence electrons, making them chemically reactive with one another. Group 1 elements, such as the alkali metals, are

excellent catalysts for the formation of ionic compounds with nonmetals.

The periodic law asserts that the properties of elements are periodic functions of their atomic numbers, which brings us to our sixth and final law. In other words, as you proceed down the periodic table, you'll notice a consistent pattern in the elements' properties.

Implications and Practical Uses

The periodic table is more than just a list of elements; it's a living, breathing tool with profound consequences for the fields of science, technology, and everyday life.

Predicting chemical properties and behaviours of elements based on their places in the periodic table is one of the primary uses of the table. This ability to foresee future events is crucial to the process of creating novel materials, comprehending chemical interactions, and creating cutting-edge technology.

2. New Elements Discovered: Vacancies in the Periodic Table Have

new elemental discoveries. Since uranium (the last naturally occurring element) was discovered, scientists have synthesised and characterised several more elements, extending our knowledge of the atomic world.

Third, Materials Science: The periodic table is essential in materials science, since it helps to direct the creation of materials with tailored qualities for certain uses. The periodic table is used as a reference while developing new materials like superconductors and semiconductors.

4. Environmental Chemistry: Chemists and environmental scientists examine the toxicity, mobility, and interactions of elements in the

environment by consulting the periodic table. Environmental policies and procedures can be better informed by this information.

5. Nuclear Physics: The study of atomic nuclei and their properties and behaviours, such as nuclear reactions and decay processes, is organised according to the periodic table.

The periodic table is a crucial learning tool for chemistry students. To help students gain a more thorough comprehension of the natural world, it gives a methodical approach to studying the components and the interactions among them.

Conclusion

The success of the periodic table is a result of human ingenuity and teamwork. It embodies the cumulative efforts of scientists over several centuries. The periodic chart is more than just a handy reference; it also represents the incredible interdependence of the substances that make up our planet.

The elements in the periodic table provide a framework for comprehending the fundamental building blocks of matter and the processes that affect our world, from the smallest atoms to the largest molecules. It allows scientists to make forecasts, find new elements, and develop materials with hitherto unattainable qualities. It's been cited as an influence by scientists and students for decades because of its role as a cornerstone in the field of chemistry education.

The periodic table will continue to be a living document as we move forward. Researchers at the atomic and subatomic levels keep pushing the limits of our knowledge of the elements and their place in the cosmos. The periodic table's continued relevance serves as a constant reminder that learning is a continuing process and that the mysteries of the universe are just waiting to be pieced together.

3.2 Properties of Elements in Groups and Periods

Elements' Periodic and Group Structures and Their Properties

The constituents of matter are represented graphically in the periodic table, a spectacular and iconic scientific creation. Rather of being a static arrangement of elements, it acts as a dynamic road map that helps us make sense of the characteristics and behaviours of those elements. The elements of the periodic table are divided into families and periods, each of which has its own unique properties and trends that shed light on the atomic nature of matter. By investigating the characteristics of substances in relation to one another and across time, we can get insight into the overarching trends and patterns that inform our perception of the natural world.

The elements in a group share certain characteristics.

The vertical columns of the periodic table are referred to as groups or families. Elements with the same atomic number tend to exhibit comparable chemical characteristics and behaviours because their valence electrons (those located in the atom's outermost energy level) also have the same number. In order to make educated guesses about the reactivity, chemical bonding, and general behaviour of elements, it is crucial to understand their properties within groups.

Group 1 consists of the alkali metals.

The alkali metals, which include lithium (Li), sodium (Na), potassium (K), and others, make up the first group of the periodic table. In the presence of water in particular, these metals tend to rapidly form compounds. As their outermost energy level contains only one valence electron, alkali metals are ready to shed this electron and transform into positively charged ions (cations). Their low density, softness, and metallic sheen make them highly desirable. Numerous industries, from the battery industry to the pharmaceutical industry, rely on alkali metals.

Alkaline Earth Metals Make Up Group 2

The alkaline earth metals are the second set, and they include elements like Mg, Ca, and Sr. The alkaline earth metals have two valence electrons, just like the alkali metals. They produce compounds with nonmetals, albeit at a lower rate than alkali metals. There are many vital biological processes that can't function without the alkaline earth metals also utilised in architecture and metalworking.

The Halogens make up Group 17.

Iodine (I), Chlorine (Cl), and Fluorine (F) make up Group 17, also called the Halogens. The strong reactivity and propensity to form compounds with metals, resulting in salts, are defining features of the halogens, a class of nonmetals. They are eager to gain electrons and transform into negatively charged ions (anions) because they contain seven valence electrons and need one more to reach a stable electron configuration. The use of halogens is essential in a variety of fields, including electronics manufacturing, photography, and disinfection.

The Noble Gases (Group 18)

Helium, neon, and argon make comprise the noble gases of Group 18. When compared to elements in other categories, noble gases stand out for being exceptionally stable and unreactive. Full valence electron shells render them chemically inert at ambient temperature and pressure. Due to their distinct qualities, noble gases find widespread application in fields as diverse as illumination (neon lights), lasers, and cryogenics.

Periods: The Elemental Energy Levels

Atomic energy levels, also known as electron shells, correspond to the periods (or rows) of the periodic table. The number of energy levels between elements in the same period is constant, but the number of subshells and electrons in each subshell is not. Insights into atomic size, electronegativity, and ionisation energy can be gained by comparing elements within their respective periods.

Atomic Dimensions and Timescales

The gradual increase or decrease in atomic size as you move through a period from left to right is a notable characteristic connected with periods. The rising number of protons in the nucleus has a greater electrostatic force on the electrons at the same energy level, leading to this trend.

Typically, atomic size decreases from left to right across a period. The reason for this is that the stronger the attraction between the nucleus and the electrons, the closer the electrons will be to the nucleus as the number of protons in the nucleus increases. The increased attraction has the effect of shrinking the atom.

In contrast, atomic size tends to grow as one descends a group in the periodic table. The accumulation of energy levels, also called electron shells, is responsible for the expansion of atoms. The radius of an atom grows when its electrons move to higher energy levels because they are now further from the nucleus.

Periods and Electronegativity

An element's electronegativity indicates how well it can draw electrons into a chemical connection. Elemental electronegativity increases towards the right side of the periodic table (the later periods), and decreases towards the left side (the earlier periods) of the table.

In general, electronegativity rises as one moves over a period from left to right. This is due to the larger nuclear charge and smaller atomic size of elements on the right side of the periodic table, both of which have a greater tendency to attract electrons. The electronegativities of the atoms on the left side of the table are lower because they contain fewer protons and are larger in size.

Energy of Ionisation and Timescales.

The ionisation energy of an atom is the amount of energy needed to strip away one of its electrons, transforming the atom into a positively charged ion. Ionisation energy, like electronegativity, follows a predictable pattern as one moves over periods and down groups.

Ionisation energy tends to rise from left to right across a period. The growing nuclear charge and shrinking atomic size are to blame for this development. It becomes more challenging to remove one electron from an atom as its number of protons increases, because the protons exert a stronger attraction on the electrons.

Ionisation energy typically drops as one moves along a clade. This is because electrons have higher energy levels farther from the nucleus as you progress down the periodic table. These periphery electrons are less strongly attracted to the nucleus electrostatically, making them more accessible for removal.

Insights from the Periodic Table

Groups and periods in the periodic table can shed light on the characteristics and behaviours of individual elements. The systematic framework provided by these patterns and trends can be applied to the study of atomic size, electronegativity, ionisation energy, and other related concepts.

Scientists and chemists can use the information provided by the periodic table to make educated guesses about the chemical and physical properties of elements, compounds, and mixtures. This ability to foresee outcomes is crucial in many areas of technology and science, including chemistry and materials research.

In addition, the periodic table is not a fixed structure but rather a dynamic resource. The ever-evolving periodic table is a reflection of humanity's never-ending drive to learn more about the world around it and the atomic and subatomic phenomena that make up its building blocks.

In conclusion, the Periodic Table is a symbol of the potential of human inquisitiveness, cooperation, and scientific study. It's crucial because it helps us connect the dots between the macroscopic and microscopic worlds, revealing the hidden secrets of the elements and their place in the greater scheme of things.

Chapter 4:
To bond chemically

4.1 Ionic Bonding

How Electrons and Ions Tango to Form Bonds

Ionic bonding is a crucial idea in the complex science of chemistry since it explains how compounds are formed and how matter behaves. When atoms share electrons, forming charged particles called ions, the ensuing chemical link is called ionic bonding. This fascinating interaction between electrons and ions is crucial in determining the characteristics of many different compounds, from simple salt to complicated mineral formations. In this investigation of ionic bonding, we will examine the underlying mechanisms of this fundamental phenomenon, as well as its role in nature and its scientific and technological applications.

Electrons and ions are the basis of ionic bonding.

Electrons, negatively charged subatomic particles that orbit the nucleus of an atom, are essential to the formation of ions. Each electron shell has a maximum capacity determined by the energy level it corresponds to. Ionic bonding relies heavily on the valence shell, the atomic nucleus's outermost energy level.

When valence shells are completely filled with electrons, atoms are at their most stable. Unfortunately, this stable conformation is not naturally attained by all atoms. Positively charged ions, or cations, are formed when elements on the left side of the periodic table, such metals, lose electrons to reach a stable, complete valence shell. The opposite is true for elements on the right side of the periodic table, such as nonmetals, which lose electrons to fill their valence shells and produce anions.

Ion Formation: Electrons in Motion

Atoms form ionic bonds because they want to have more stable electron configurations. The production of ions with opposite charges results from this process, which requires the transfer of electrons from one atom to another. Let's have a look at the moves in this electronic tango:

First, cations are formed when a metal's valence shell is depleted and it loses electrons to fill it up to a stable level. The loss of one or more electrons from a metal atom converts it to a positively charged cation. The outermost shell of sodium (Na) atoms has one valence electron. The Na+ ion is formed when sodium loses one electron.

Anions are formed when a nonmetal's valence shell is nearly full but needs a few more electrons to reach a stable state, as discussed in (2). An anion is a negatively charged ion formed when a nonmetal atom receives an electron or more. In contrast, chlorine (Cl) only possesses seven and hence needs one more valence electron to complete its valence shell. Chlorine, after gaining an electron, becomes the Cl ion.

Third, Electrostatic Attraction: Ions and cations are drawn to each other by electrostatic forces after they have produced. Strong attraction exists between ions with opposite charges, leading to the formation of ionic compounds.

Ionic compounds are formed when ions bond to each other.

Ionic compounds, or salts, are the result of the electrostatic attraction between cations and anions. Ionic bonding gives these molecules their unique characteristics:

Ionic compounds frequently take on a crystalline form, where the ions are grouped in a repeating pattern known as a crystal lattice. The rigidity and brittleness of the compounds can be attributed in part to their orderly arrangement.

The high melting and boiling temperatures of ionic compounds are a result of the strong electrostatic interactions between ions, which necessitate a great deal of energy to break the bonds and transform the solid into a liquid or gas.

Thirdly, ionic substances do not conduct electricity in the solid state because the ions are not free to move around the crystal lattice. When melted or dissolved in water, however, the ions are free to travel and carry electric charge, making the materials great conductors of electricity.

4. Solubility: Many ionic chemicals dissolve and create aqueous solutions in water because the polar water molecules may enclose and separate the ions.

The Most Frequently Encountered Ionic Compounds

There are several uses for the common ionic chemicals found in nature. Ionic compounds contain several common substances, such as:

The most well-known ionic chemical is probably sodium chloride (NaCl), or table salt. It is made up of a crystal lattice of sodium cations (Na^+) and chloride anions (Cl^-). Seasoning, food preservation, and numerous industrial uses are just some of salt's many applications.

Limestone, chalk, and marble are all examples of calcium carbonate's natural incarnations, and it goes by the chemical formula $CaCO_3$. It is also the main ingredient in coral, shells, and hard water deposits.

Potassium nitrate (KNO3), often known as saltpetre, has a number of applications such as a fertiliser additive, a component of fireworks, and a food preservative cure.

Epsom salt, a hydrate of magnesium sulphate, is commonly used for its medicinal effects in bath salts, making it the fourth ingredient on the list. It's also used as a drying agent in chemistry labs and in agriculture.

Utilisation of Ionic Substances

Ionic compounds are extremely important, and not just because they are used as table salt. They can be used in several contexts as as

Analytical chemistry relies heavily on ionic chemicals, both for qualitative and quantitative analysis, making them an important aspect of the field. It is usual practise to determine the identity and concentration of ions in a solution by precipitation reactions that result in the creation of insoluble ionic compounds.

Second, several ionic chemicals are used in medicine, either as therapeutics or as markers for disease. Antacids, for instance, typically include ionic substances like aluminium hydroxide (Al(OH)3) and magnesium hydroxide (Mg(OH)2).

3. Metallurgy: Ionic chemicals, such as calcium oxide (CaO) and sodium cyanide (NaCN), are commonly used as fluxes and reagents in the metallurgical process of extracting metals from their ores.

4. Environmental research: It is essential in environmental research to have a firm grasp on how ionic substances behave when introduced to soil and water. Ion mobility and solubility influence plant nutrient availability and water quality.

5. Energy Storage: Ionic chemicals are utilised in electrolytes for batteries and supercapacitors, among other energy storage

technologies. Ionic mobility, which produces electrical energy, is made possible by these chemicals.

Ionic liquids, which are salts in their liquid form, are utilised as green solvents and catalysts in a wide variety of chemical reactions, including those in the pharmaceutical and petrochemical sectors.

Directions for the Future and Current Challenges

Ionic compounds are crucial to our understanding of chemistry and have many practical applications, but they also present certain difficulties. The mining and extraction of ionic compound resources has a significant influence on the environment. Research and development are ongoing in the fields of sustainable practises and alternative materials.

And research into ionic chemicals and bonding continues to thrive. Researchers are constantly looking for new ionic materials to study.

 special qualities, such the adaptability of ionic liquids to a variety of uses.In sum: The Dance Goes OnIonic bonding, which is propelled by electron exchange and the creation of ions, is a fundamental process that determines the nature of numerous compounds. Ionic compounds play a crucial role in our knowledge of matter and its behaviour, from the common table salt used to season food to the complex materials employed in cutting-edge technologies.

Electron and ion dances will continue to unfurl as science and technology progress, revealing previously unimaginable substances and uses. This complex dance of chemistry contains not just the wonders of nature but also the untapped potential for new knowledge that has inspired generations of scientists and scholars. Ionic bonding is a monument to the beauty and relevance of the natural world and the human drive for discovery and improvement.

4.2 Covalent Bonding

Harmony of Shared Electrons in Covalent Bonding

Covalent bonding, which underlies the creation of molecules, is an intriguing and essential idea in chemistry. It's a delicate dance of electrons, where atoms join together and trade off their outer electrons to form a stable network. The chemistry of life, the creation of compounds, and the complexity of matter are all driven by covalent bonds, which are common in nature. The mechanics of covalent bonding, its significance in various fields, and its role in forming our environment will all be investigated in this article.

Electrons and valence shells, the building blocks of covalent bonds.

Covalent bonding requires knowledge of electrons and the atomic idea of valence shells. Electrons are negatively charged particles that have their own energy levels, or "shells," as they orbit the nucleus of an atom. Covalent bonding relies heavily on the outermost shell, the valence shell.

When valence shells are completely filled with electrons, atoms are at their most stable. The chemical properties and reactivity of an atom are determined by its valence electron count. Chemical characteristics of elements are generally similar across those in the same group of the periodic table because of shared valence electron configurations.

Shared electrons are the key of covalent bonding.

The need for atoms to achieve a stable electron configuration drives them to share electrons with other atoms, a process known as covalent bonding. Atoms bond through this intricate dance of shared electrons to form molecules. Let's have a look at each stage of this complicated procedure:

A covalent bond involves the sharing of electrons between two or more atoms in order to create a more stable electronic arrangement. A covalent link, often called a chemical bond, is the region of high electron density that forms when electrons are shared between atoms.

2. Electron Pair: Two atoms form a covalent connection by giving and receiving an electron pair. The shared pair of electrons between the atoms acts as a connection between the atoms.

3. Molecular Structure: The number and spatial orientation of bonds between atoms in a covalent molecule influence the arrangement of those atoms. The molecular architectures of covalent compounds can vary greatly, from linear and tetrahedral to planar and beyond.

4. Single, Double, and Triple Bonds: Covalent bonds are categorised as single, double, or triple depending on the number of shared electron pairs. It takes one pair of electrons to form a single bond (like H2), two pairs (like O2), and three pairs (like N2) to form a double or triple bond.

The electronegativity (the tendency to attract electrons) of the atoms involved determines whether a covalent bond is polar or nonpolar. When there is a large disparity in electronegativity between two atoms, the resulting bond is polar, with one atom carrying a partial negative charge and the other a partial positive one. The electrons in nonpolar covalent bonds are shared between the bonded molecules.

Covalent compounds' characteristics

Because of the unique nature of covalent bonding, molecular compounds (also known as covalent compounds) exhibit a number of distinctive characteristics.

1. Lower Melting and Boiling values: Compared to ionic compounds, covalent compounds often have lower melting and boiling values.

The reason for this is that in covalent compounds, the intermolecular forces are not as strong as the electrostatic forces in ionic compounds.

Solubility 2: Many covalent compounds can dissolve in benzene and other nonpolar solvents since they are themselves nonpolar molecules. However, they typically cannot dissolve in nonpolar liquids.

Since covalent compounds lack ions and free-moving electrons, they do not conduct electricity in either the solid or liquid state. However, under certain conditions, some covalent compounds can transmit electricity while dissolved in water or even in a pure solid state.

Covalent substances can take on many different forms, including gases (like oxygen and nitrogen), liquids (like water and ethanol), and solids (like sugar and iodine).

Why Covalent Bonds Are So Important

Covalent bonds have far-reaching ramifications in many different areas and are hence of great importance in the natural world:

Covalent bonding form the basis of all biochemical processes, according to first-year biology textbooks. Covalent links unite the DNA, proteins, and carbohydrates that make up all living things. Covalent bonding are necessary for the catalytic actions of enzymes, which are pivotal in virtually all biological processes.

2. Pharmaceutics: Pharmaceutical development requires knowledge of covalent bond chemistry. In order to be effective, medications must first create covalent connections with their intended targets within the body.

Third, Materials Science, where new materials with tailored properties are conceived and developed, relies heavily on covalent compounds. Polymers are a type of big molecule that is created by covalent connections and can be found in a wide variety of plastics, textiles, and other commonplace items.

4. Environmental Science: In this field, a firm grasp of the chemistry underlying covalent molecules is essential. It's useful for researching how toxins break down in the environment and what chemicals ecosystems use to function.

5. Chemical Industry: Many chemicals, from pharmaceuticals and agrochemicals to creating specialised compounds, are synthesised using the principles of covalent bonding.

Implications for Future Research

Although scientists have a good handle on how covalent bonds work, there is still plenty to learn about them. Covalent bonding principles are driving the discovery of novel compounds and materials with interesting characteristics. The study of covalent bonds under extreme conditions, such as high pressures and temperatures, the creation of innovative materials with customised features, and other similar tasks all present difficulties.The Finale of Our Shared Electron SymphonyThe production of numerous molecules in nature is predicated on covalent bonding, the cornerstone of chemistry that involves a complicated dance of shared electrons. It's the stuff of life, the stuff of substance, and the stuff of invention. Covalent bonds have profound implications for our knowledge of the cosmos, from the smallest diatomic molecules to the largest biological cromolecules.Covalent bonding, with its shared electron symphony, will continue to be at the vanguard of discovery as we learn more about the natural world and make technological advances. It's proof that the subatomic world is just as beautiful as the macroscopic one, and that humans will never stop seeking to learn more about the universe and the laws that govern it.

Chapter 5:
Involvement in Reactions

5.1 Types of Chemical Reactions

Different Categories of Chemical Reactions: How Matter Is Transformed

The constant transformation of our environment is the result of chemical processes. They are in charge of the chemical reactions that keep the biosphere alive and the technological systems running. To forecast, manage, and take advantage of these transformations, it is essential to have a firm grasp of the different kinds of chemical reactions that can occur. We will examine the major classes of chemical processes, what makes them unique, and how they are used in the natural and artificial worlds.

The Concept of Chemical Reactions

When two or more substances with distinct chemical characteristics (reactants) combine, a chemical reaction takes place. Chemical bonds between atoms and molecules are broken and formed during these transitions. The overall mass and energy of a system do not change during a chemical reaction because of the laws of conservation of mass and energy.

Important Groups of Reactions in Chemistry

Different types of chemical reactions are distinguished by the properties they exhibit and the modifications they cause to the chemical structure of substances. There are primarily two categories of chemical reactions:

Synthesis Reactions, or Combination Reactions, 1. Multiple reactants are brought together to generate a single product in combination reactions. A + B = AB, where A and B are the reactants and AB is the result, is a common symbolic representation of such reactions. Two hydrogens and two oxygens make two hydrogen dioxides and two hydrogen oxides, or water.

Reactions that decompose a chemical into two or more simpler compounds are called decomposition reactions. Decomposition reactions follow the formula AB = A + B. Hydrogen peroxide, for instance, can be broken down into water and oxygen via the chemical equation $2H_2O_2$ $2H_2O + O_2$.

Third, Displacement Reactions (Single Replacement Reactions): One element or ion replaces another in a compound during single replacement reactions. A + BC AC + B is the general equation for a single-replacement reaction. For instance, zinc (Zn) displaces hydrogen (H2) in the reaction zinc (Zn) and hydrochloric acid (HCl) to generate zinc chloride (ZnCl2): $Zn + 2HCl$ $ZnCl_2 + H_2$.

Double-replacement (or synthesis) reactions The production of two new compounds is the consequence of an ion exchange between two compounds in a double replacement reaction. AB + CD AD + CB is the universal equation for the double replacement reaction. One such reaction is the formation of silver chloride (AgCl) and sodium nitrate ($NaNO_3$) from sodium chloride (NaCl) and silver nitrate ($AgNO_3$), respectively.

Five, Neutralisation Reactions (Acid-Base Reactions): The transfer of a proton (H^+ ion) from an acid to a base results in the formation of water and a salt in a process known as an acid-base reaction. Acid and bases react with one another to produce water and salt. Hydrochloric acid (HCl) and sodium hydroxide (NaOH) react to produce water (H_2O) and sodium chloride (NaCl), for instance.

Oxidation-Reduction Reactions (also known as Redox Reactions): The electrons in a redox reaction are moved from one reactant to another. One material loses electrons through oxidation, whereas another gains them through reduction. These reactions are essential in electron transport and energy production. Hydrogen (H2) burns in the presence of oxygen (O2) to produce water (H2O) as an illustration: $2H_2 + O_2 \rightarrow 2H_2O$.

Chemical Equation Balancing

The proper representation of chemical reactions requires balancing chemical equations. According to the principle of mass conservation, both sides of the equation must have the same number of atoms of each element. To check that the total number of atoms of each element is the same on both sides of an equation, coefficients (whole numbers) are added before the chemical formulas.

Take the imbalanced equation for the combustion of methane (CH4) in oxygen (O2) as an illustration. CH4 + O2 CO2 + H2O. Coefficients are added until the scales are even: The reaction between CH4 and 2O2 produces CO2 and 2H2O. The number of carbon, hydrogen, and oxygen atoms on each side of the equation is now equal.

Implications and Practical UsesThere are many contexts in which knowledge of chemical reaction types is crucial:

First, the Chemical Industry relies heavily on chemical reactions in order to produce goods such as Pharmaceuticals, Fertilisers, Plastics, and Fuels.

2. Environmental Science: The study of chemical processes, such as pollutant degradation, nutrient cycling, and the chemistry of natural ecosystems, requires an understanding of chemical interactions. The development and production of pharmaceuticals that target specific biochemical pathways in the human body requires an understanding of chemical interactions, which is the focus of pharmaceutical research.

4. Energy Production: Combustion and nuclear reactions are just two examples of energy production systems that rely on chemical reactions that release energy as heat or electricity.

5. Materials Science: Polymers, composites, and sophisticated ceramics, among others, are designed and synthesised with specific qualities by chemical reactions.

6. Biological Processes: The chemical reactions that support the functioning of living organisms include photosynthesis, cellular respiration, and enzymatic reactions.Implications for Future Research Extensive study and new developments have been made in the field of chemical reactions. To enhance reaction efficiency, selectivity, and sustainability, scientists investigate novel catalysts, reaction conditions, and materials. Studies in "green chemistry," for example, aim to cut down on waste and energy usage in chemical production.

High-pressure and high-temperature reactions are also being studied at an increasing rate. The results of these studies can be used to improve energy generation, create new materials, and learn more about the inner workings of the Earth.Finishing Up: Matter's Amazing ChangesThe natural world and human civilization are both propelled forward by chemical reactions in their many forms.scientific and technological domain. They are the rules that determine how life works, how new materials are made, and how energy is transferred to keep the world running.

As we learn more about how chemicals interact, we can use that knowledge to address previously intractable problems. Learning about these interactions not only deepens our comprehension of the natural world, but also gives us new tools for engineering, innovation, and raising standards of living everywhere. Material changes, as shown by various chemical reactions, continue to attest to the dynamic character of science and its infinite potential for discovery and improvement.

5.2 Balancing Chemical Equations

The Crucial Skill of Balancing Chemical Equations

Understanding chemical processes requires mastery of the fundamental ability of balancing chemical equations. These simple mathematical equations reveal the identities and amounts of components involved in the transformation of reactants into products. By ensuring that the total mass of reactants and products are equal, balancing chemical equations upholds the law of conservation of mass. In this investigation of chemical equation balancing, we will investigate the rationale for this crucial ability, investigate the procedures for balancing equations, and analyse its relevance in many scientific and technological contexts.

Chemical equations have been called "the language of chemistry."

Chemical reactions are represented symbolically by chemical equations. They offer a condensed means of communicating the reactants, products, and stoichiometry (the mole ratios of each item involved) of a reaction. When the number of atoms of each element in the reactant and the number of atoms of the same element in the product are both the same, we have a balanced chemical equation.

When methane (CH_4) and oxygen (O_2) are burned, carbon dioxide (CO_2) and water (H_2O) are produced.

CO_2 and water are produced when oxygen is added to CH_4. This equation does a good job of describing the reaction as a whole, however it is not balanced. Adjusting the coefficients (whole numbers) in front of the chemical formulas to achieve a balance is necessary to uphold the law of conservation of mass.

The Procedure for Balancing Chemical Equations

The coefficients of the reactants and the products must be adjusted so that the total number of atoms of each element in both the reactants and the products are identical. The following are the procedures for achieving chemical equilibrium:

First, Note the Uneven Equation: To get started, just write down the chemical equation for the reaction. Be sure to list all the constituents and end-products.

2. Tally the Number of Atoms on Both Sides of the Equation: For each element, tally the atomic counts on both sides of the equation. Take the items that are unique to both sides as a starting point.

3. Trace the Uneven Components: Find the elements where the reactant and product have different atomic counts. All of these parts should be in harmony with one another.

The coefficients of the chemical formulas in the equation must be adjusted to bring the elements that appear in only one compound on each side into balance. The formulas need to have full numbers added to them for this to work.
Recount the atoms of each element to ensure mathematical accuracy after making changes to the coefficients. If the elements are not in harmony, the process of modifying the coefficients must be repeated.

Number six: Use the Lowest Whole Numbers: Use the lowest whole numbers as coefficients to achieve a balanced equation. This guarantees an accurate depiction of the reaction's stoichiometry.

7. Special circumstances: It may be essential to alter numerous coefficients to establish balance in certain circumstances, especially with complex reactions or reactions involving polyatomic ions.

Let's use these procedures to ignite methane:
CO_2 and water are produced when oxygen is added to CH_4.

Atomic Numbers:

In the first column (reactants):
Carbon (C) Count: 1
H4 = Hydrogen
Oxygen (O) Count: 2 (O2 Count)

Products are displayed on the right.
Carbon (C) Count: 1
Oxygen (O): 3 (from CO2 and H2O) - Hydrogen (H): 2 (from H2O)

Spotting Uneven Components:

The ratio of carbon to hydrogen is off.

Coefficient Adjustment

On the product side, we adjust for carbon by adding a coefficient of 1 to CO2:

CH4 and O2 combine to form carbon dioxide and water vapour.

The carbon cycle has been reset.

The hydrogen equilibrium comes next. The left side has four hydrogen atoms, while the right side contains only two. To counteract this, we multiply H2O by a factor of 2 on the product side:

CO2 and water vapour are produced when CH4 is exposed to oxygen.

Repetition and Verification:
We re-count the atoms after making the necessary changes to the coefficients:

In the first column (reactants):
Carbon (C) Count: 1
H4 = Hydrogen
Oxygen (O) Count: 2 (O2 Count)

Products are displayed on the right.
Carbon (C) Count: 1
4 hydrogen atoms (H) (2 H from each H2O molecule)
Number of Oxygen (O) atoms: 4 (2 from CO2 and 2 from H2O).

The equation now stands, with all atoms in equilibrium, as follows:

It can be written as:

There are an equal number of atoms of each element on both sides of this equation, therefore it appropriately depicts the burning of methane.

Importance of Obtaining a Correct Chemical Formula
The ability to balance chemical equations is fundamental and has far-reaching implications in many fields of science and industry.
One must be able to balance equations in order to describe chemical reactions and comprehend the transformation of reactants into products.

2. Stoichiometry: The stoichiometric connections between reactants and products are provided by balanced equations, allowing scientists to determine the amounts of chemicals needed for a reaction.

3. Chemical Synthesis: Balancing equations is crucial in chemical synthesis when planning and optimising processes to produce desired products.
4. Chemical Analysis: In analytical chemistry, concentrations of chemicals in a sample are calculated using balanced equations that take into account the amounts of reactants and products.

5. Environmental Chemistry: In order to analyse pollutant transformations, degradation processes, and the impact of chemical reactions on ecosystems, a firm grasp of balanced equations is essential.

Using balanced equations, chemical engineers plan and manage chemical processes like those used to make things like fuel, medicine, and other materials.

Implications for Future Research
Chemical equation balance is a fundamental ability, although it can get tricky for complex reactions with many reactants and products. Computational chemists and chemical informaticians are working to automate the task of balancing equations and forecasting reaction outcomes by using software tools and algorithms. The instruments can be used in the pharmaceutical industry, materials research, and reaction optimisation.

Research into reaction mechanisms and kinetics is another area that is still developing. In order to create more effective and selective chemical processes, scientists study the finer points of chemical interactions at the molecular level.

reactions.

Finally, in Chemistry, we Have Reached Equilibrium

Chemical equation balancing is more than just a mathematical exercise; it is essential to understanding the complex material changes that characterise chemistry. It helps us convey the essence of chemical reactions, make accurate predictions, and design efficient systems. The capacity to balance chemical equations is crucial to our pursuit of understanding, manipulating, and harnessing the power of chemical reactions for the benefit of science and society at all levels of investigation, from the most basic to the most applied.

Chapter 6:
Bases and Acids

6.1 Properties of Acids and Bases

The Chemistry Behind Salty and Sour Flavours: Acid and Base Properties

In chemistry, acids and bases are two types of fundamental chemicals that play essential roles in determining how matter behaves. Natural events, chemical reactions, and industrial operations all rely on an appreciation of their qualities. In this investigation of acid and basic qualities, we will examine their unique attributes, chemical behaviour, everyday relevance, and scientific and technological uses.

Acids and Bases: A First Course

Substances belonging to the acidic and basic groups exhibit polar opposite properties:

To begin, we have Acids, which are compounds that give up their protons (H+ ions) to other molecules. The presence of hydrogen ions in their chemical formulas, along with their sour flavour and tendency to dye blue litmus paper red, distinguish them as acids. Hydrochloric acid (HCl), sulfuric acid (H2SO4), and citric acid (found in citrus fruits) are all examples of acids.

Bases, on the other hand, are compounds that donate hydroxide ions (OH) or take protons (H+ ions) from other substances. They'll turn red litmus paper blue, have a bitter flavour, and feel slick to the touch. Sodium hydroxide (NaOH), ammonia (NH3), and calcium hydroxide (Ca(OH)2) are all examples of common bases.

Acid Properties

A number of unique characteristics distinguish acids different from other substances:

First, a sour flavour; acidic things, like lemon juice and vinegar, have a sour flavour. However, due to potential risks, it is not advised to taste chemicals.

Acids react with metals like zinc and magnesium, releasing hydrogen gas (H2) in the process. One reaction produces zinc chloride (ZnCl2) and hydrogen gas from hydrochloric acid (HCl) and zinc, respectively.

In order to create ZnCl2 and H2 gas, HCl must be added to zinc.

Thirdly, Corrosive Properties: Concentrated acids can be quite corrosive, damaging or dissolving objects like metals and organic stuff. This quality is put to use in numerous commercial contexts, most notably in the metal cleaning and pickling industries.

Fourth, acids have electrolyte properties, which means that they conduct electricity when dissolved in water. This is because in water they break apart into ions (H+ and anions).

Fifth, some indicators will shift colours when exposed to acids. For instance, they alter the hue of phenolphthalein from colourless to pink and cause blue litmus paper to turn red.

6. pH 7: Acids have pH values below 7 on the 0–14 pH scale. An acid with a lower pH is more acidic than one with a higher pH.

7. Neutralisation: A neutralisation reaction occurs when an acid and a base combine to produce a salt and water. Multiple uses rely on this process, including antacids for gastrointestinal distress.

Base Characteristics

In addition to being chemically distinct, bases have the following characteristics:

Baking soda (sodium bicarbonate) and other bases have a bitter flavour because of this property. However, much like acid, chemical tasting is not recommended.

Two, Slippery Feel: Bases have a soapy or slick sensation when touched. Soaps and detergents have this characteristic, which is easily noticed by anyone who has used them.

Thirdly, bases undergo saponification when they come into contact with oils and fats. Soap and glycerol are created through the hydrolysis of fats and oils using a base (such as sodium hydroxide) in the soap-making process.

Since bases contain hydroxide ions (OH), they also have the electrolyte properties of conducting electricity when dissolved in water.

The colour of certain indicators is altered when a base is used. They can, for instance, alter the hue of phenolphthalein from colourless to pink or cause red litmus paper to turn blue.

Sixth, pH Greater Than 7: Bases have a pH greater than 7. If the pH value is high, the base is strong, and if it is low, the base is weak.

Whenever a base comes into contact with an acid, a neutralisation reaction takes place. Two byproducts of this reaction are water and a salt.

Daily Life Importance of Acids and Bases

There are many aspects of our daily life that are affected by acids and bases:

Hydrochloric acid (HCl) in the stomach is an essential component of the digestive process. It creates an acidic environment that is lethal to dangerous bacteria and aids in the breakdown of proteins.

2. Cleaning Products: Bases (such as ammonia and sodium hydroxide) are commonly found in household cleaning solutions and aid in the dissolution of grime, grease, and stains. Laundry detergents rely on bases as well.

Thirdly, Food and Beverages: Acids and bases are present in many foods and beverages and can alter their flavour and shelf life. Citrus fruits are a good source of citric acid, while lactic acid is created during the cheesemaking process.

Acids and bases are utilised in a wide variety of medicines and pharmaceuticals. Acid reflux and indigestion can be alleviated with the help of antacids, which include bases to neutralise the stomach's excess acid.

In agriculture, acids and bases are used to control soil pH, which in turn affects plant growth and harvests. If they have acidic soil, farmers might apply lime (a base) to make it more alkaline.

Impact on the Environment Number Six: Acid rain is a major problem because of emissions of sulphur dioxide (SO_2) and nitrogen oxides (NOx) into the atmosphere. Ecosystems, buildings, and water sources are all under risk.

Acids and Bases in Everyday Life

Numerous industries and uses put acid and basic qualities to good use.

One example of chemical manufacturing is the making of fertilisers, medicines, and polymers, all of which rely on acids and bases as catalysts and reagents.

The pH of water is adjusted in water treatment facilities using bases like sodium hydroxide (NaOH), ensuring that the water is suitable for human consumption.

Acids are used in metal cleaning and etching procedures, while bases are put to use in metal refining and extraction, as discussed in (3)Metallurgy.

Acids and bases are common food additives used to improve flavour, extend shelf life, and modify the pH of foods.

Acids and bases are indispensable in titrations and pH measurements, two of the most common analytical procedures used in the laboratory.

Battery electrolytes are typically either acidic or basic solutions that allow ions to move and electrical energy to be generated.

Implications for Future Research
While scientists have a good grasp of acids and bases and their characteristics, they continue to investigate greener ways of doing things. The goal of green chemistry projects is to

 to devise strategies for decreasing reliance on potentially harmful acids and bases, cutting down on waste, and maximising chemical processes' energy efficiency.

In addition, studies investigate the extreme conditions under which superacids (extremely strong acids) and superbases (extremely strong bases) behave, shedding light on their possible uses in fields such as catalysis and materials science.

Sour and Bitter: The Chemistry of Flavour
Understanding the chemical world and our ability to alter and control chemical processes relies heavily on our knowledge of acids and

bases and their unique tastes, textures, and chemical behaviours. Acids and bases are fundamental to a vast array of phenomena and applications, from the chemistry of our digestive systems to the industrial processes that power the contemporary world.

The importance of acids and bases will increase as our knowledge and studies improve. A more sustainable and efficient world will be possible because to their contributions to green chemistry, sustainable technologies, and cutting-edge materials. Acids and bases, and the chemistry of sour and bitter they embody, are an indelible and fundamental part of our scientific and everyday life.

6.2 pH Scale

What the pH Scale Reveals About Acidity and Alkalinity

The pH scale is a strong instrument for measuring and comprehending the acidity or alkalinity of things, and it is a cornerstone idea in chemistry. Understanding the concentration of hydrogen ions (H+) in a solution, which is measured on a logarithmic scale, is useful for many different types of scientific, industrial, and scholarly endeavours. Learn more about the history, definition, significance, and practical applications of the pH scale, as well as its far-reaching effects in the scientific and technological communities, in this in-depth analysis.

The pH Scale's Historical Roots

In the early 20th century, Danish biochemist Sren Peder Lauritz Srensen invented the pH scale. Srensen created the scale to standardise the expression of acidity and alkalinity for use in his studies of enzymes and proteins at the Carlsberg Laboratory in Copenhagen, Denmark. He called his scale "pH," where "p" stands for the German word for "power," "potenz," and "H" is the chemical symbol for hydrogen.

The initial definition of the pH scale was the negative logarithm (base 10) of the concentration of hydrogen ions:

$$pH = -\log(H+)$$

The pH scale, developed by Sorensen, simplified the process of quantifying and conveying information about the acidity or alkalinity of solutions.

Knowing How to Use the pH Scale

The neutral point, or pH 7, is located in the midpoint of the pH scale, which runs from 0 to 14. Acidic solutions have a pH value below 7, while alkaline (basic) solutions have a pH value over 7. When the hydrogen ion concentration (H+) and hydroxide ion concentration (OH) in a solution are both 7, the solution is considered to be neutral.

Acidic (pH 7) Solutions: The concentration of hydrogen ions (H+) is greater than that of hydroxide ions (OH) in acidic liquids. The higher the acidity, the lower the pH value. A solution with a pH of 3 is more acidic than one with a pH of 5, as an illustration.

- Alkaline (Basic) Solutions (pH > 7) The concentration of hydroxide ions (OH) exceeds that of hydrogen ions (H+) in basic solutions. The more alkaline a solution is, the higher its pH value. An alkaline solution, such as one with a pH value of 10, is more so than an acidic one, such as one with a pH value of 8.

pH 7 Neutral Solutions: The concentration of hydrogen ions (H+) and hydroxide ions (OH) are both zero in neutral solutions. The pH of pure water at 25 degrees Celsius is 7, making it a neutral solution.

The pH Scale

A pH metre or pH indicator paper (pH paper) can be used to determine a solution's pH value. Accurate readings of the voltage produced by a pH electrode in a solution can be obtained with the help of a pH metre. The pH level is determined by converting the voltage.

In contrast, pH indicator paper is infused with substances that alter their hue in response to shifts in pH. One can roughly determine the pH of a solution by observing its colour shift and comparing it to a standard chart. Litmus paper, phenolphthalein, and bromothymol blue are some of the most often used indicators of pH.

Role of the pH Scale in Everyday Life

The pH scale is a useful resource for many fields of study and everyday life.

Reaction speeds, product generation, and reactant behaviour are all significantly affected by pH in chemical processes (1). In both chemistry and biology, acid-base reactions play a crucial role.

In the field of environmental science, pH is an important metric since it has a direct impact on the well-being of ecosystems and aquatic organisms. It measures the acidity of lakes and rivers to determine the extent of pollution and to track changes over time.

Thirdly, agriculture relies heavily on soil pH since it determines how easily plants can absorb nutrients. Raising crop yields and maximising fertiliser efficiency through adjusting soil pH.

In the fields of medicine and biology, the management of pH plays a crucial role in the upkeep of physiological systems. The blood's pH, for instance, is strictly controlled to ensure that enzymes and metabolic pathways work as they should.

pH has an effect on the flavour, texture, and even safety of food and beverages. It plays a vital role in the processes of preserving food, fermenting it, and creating new foods.

The pH Scale in Everyday Life

Numerous fields make use of the pH scale in various ways:

One of the ways that drinking water is made safe and up to code is through the use of pH controls in water treatment plants. Pipe corrosion can be avoided and disinfection processes guaranteed by adjusting the pH.

Second, agriculture relies heavily on accurate results from soil pH tests to calculate lime needs and maximise plant nutrition. It's useful for farmers to have accurate data when deciding how much fertiliser to use and what crops to grow.

The comfort of swimmers and the efficacy of pool sanitizers depend on keeping pool water at a consistent pH level.

4. Medical Diagnostics: The acidity or alkalinity of biological fluids like blood and urine can be determined by measuring their pH. Condition indicators include abnormal pH levels.

In order to maximise the removal of contaminants and guarantee conformity with environmental standards, proper pH control is critical in the wastewater treatment process.

Keeping an eye on and controlling pH is essential in the food processing industry for the sake of quality, safety, and shelf life. Pickling and canning are two examples of acidic preservation procedures.

Implications for Future Research

While the idea of a pH scale is not new, researchers are always working to perfect more precise and flexible pH testing instruments. Miniaturised and portable pH sensors for use in fields as diverse as environmental monitoring and medical diagnostics have become a reality because to advances in nanotechnology and microfabrication.

Furthermore, studies investigate pH regulation's effects on health and disease, as well as the pH dynamics of biological systems. Drug design and individual treatment plans can benefit greatly from research on the pH-dependent behaviour of biological entities like enzymes and proteins.

pH Has Power, A Final Thought

Our understanding of chemical processes and their effects on the natural world has been revolutionised by the pH scale, which provides a simple yet powerful logarithmic depiction of acidity and alkalinity. The behaviour of matter and life is profoundly influenced by pH, both in the controlled conditions of labs and the complex ecosystems of our planet.

Medical, agricultural, and environmental sciences, among others, will all be impacted by the pH scale as scientists continue to unlock the mysteries of pH-dependent events. The incredible ability to measure, analyse, and manage acidity and alkalinity in the world around us may be found in this logarithmic path from highly acidic to highly alkaline.

Chapter 7:
Thermodynamics in Chemistry

7.1 Laws of Thermodynamics

Principles of Energy and Matter: The Laws of Thermodynamics

The behaviour of energy and matter in the universe is governed by a set of fundamental principles known as the laws of thermodynamics. These rules lay the groundwork for comprehending anything from petrol behaviour and engine efficiency to biological processes and the ultimate fate of the universe. The four laws of thermodynamics will be examined in detail, as will their evolution, historical applications, and practical uses, as well as their far-reaching consequences in a wide range of scientific fields.

Evolution of Thermodynamics Through Time

The study of heat and its effects on matter led to the birth of the scientific field of thermodynamics, which has its origins in the 17th century. However, it wasn't until the 19th century that thermodynamics became a recognised subfield of physics thanks to the efforts of people like Sadi Carnot, Rudolf Clausius, and Lord Kelvin.

Law of thermal equilibrium (sometimes known as the Zeroth Law of Thermodynamics): Even though it wasn't one of the "big three," the Zeroth Law is essential to thermodynamics nonetheless. It defines temperature and the mutable characteristic of thermal equilibrium. According to this principle, if two systems are in thermal equilibrium with a third system, then they are also in thermal equilibrium with each other. This equation provided the theoretical basis for the study of temperature and the creation of temperature scales.

The First Law of Thermodynamics states that [[[[[[energy]] must be conserved]]; Energy, according to the First Law, often known as the

Law of Energy Conservation, cannot be created or destroyed; it can only be transformed. The principle of energy conservation is another name for this law. That is to say, in a closed system, the sum of all energies does not change.

Law of entropy, or the Second Law of Thermodynamics, states that: Entropy, defined by the Second Law as "a measure of the disorder or randomness of a system," is first introduced. It states that an isolated system's overall entropy will always increase over time during any energy transfer or change. It essentially establishes the course of nature, with an emphasis on the permanence of some changes.

Law of Absolute Zero (or the Third Law of Thermodynamics): The Third Law defines 0 degrees Celsius as the absolute lowest temperature conceivable. It claims that entropy tends to zero as a system cools to zero degrees Celsius. The study of low-temperature physics and the properties of matter close to absolute zero relies heavily on this law.

Recognising the Thermodynamic Principle

Let's take a closer look at the four fundamental principles of thermodynamics:

First, the Zeroth Law of Thermodynamics: Comparable to the idea of thermal equilibrium is the Zeroth Law. Thermal equilibrium between two things A and B implies that the temperatures of both A and B are the same with respect to a third object C. The establishment of the Celsius and Fahrenheit temperature scales is directly attributable to this equation, which provides an objective basis for defining and measuring temperature.

The First Law of Thermodynamics (Thermodynamic Energy Conservation) states: According to the First Law, energy can only be transformed from one form to another; it cannot be created or destroyed. The consequences of this principle are extensive. In a heat engine (such an internal combustion engine), for instance, the energy released as fuel burns is transformed into mechanical work and waste heat. In a chemical reaction, the energy held in atoms and molecules is released as heat and mechanical work. The concept that energy is a conserved quantity is established in the First Law, which lays the groundwork for the study of thermodynamic processes.

Third, Entropy and Irreversibility in the Second Law of Thermodynamics: The idea of entropy, which quantifies the degree of disorder in a system, is introduced in the Second Law. The overall entropy of a closed system is assumed to rise with time in any natural process. This law explains why a variety of natural processes, from ice melting to gas diffusion, tend to progress from more ordered to more chaotic states. In addition, it explains what it means for a process to be irreversible if it increases entropy. Because doing so would decrease the egg's entropy, for instance, unscrambling it is physically impossible.

Fourth Law of Thermodynamics (Entropy and Absolute Zero): The Third Law defines 0 degrees Celsius as the point at which a system has the least amount of energy. As a system cools to zero, its entropy decreases until it is equal to zero. The study of superconductivity and superfluidity, which occur at extremely low temperatures, rely heavily on this equation. It also serves to stress how theoretically impossible it is to reach absolute zero.
Thermodynamics' Useful Practical Applications

The rules of thermodynamics have wide-ranging practical and academic implications:Thermodynamics is fundamental to the field of engineering and is used extensively in the creation and maintenance of mechanical devices such as engines, power plants, refrigeration systems, and industrial production methods. Thermodynamic rinciples are used by engineers to enhance functionality and effectiveness.

2. Chemistry: Thermodynamics is fundamental to the study of chemical reactions, providing insight into the spontaneity, equilibrium, and energy changes that characterise these processes. It helps in the creation of new materials and the design of chemical processes.

Thermodynamics has many uses in physics, from investigating the features of black holes and the enlargement of the universe to better comprehending the behaviour of gases and phase transitions. Entropy is a key concept in both quantum physics and statistical mechanics.

4. Biology: Living beings and cells are subject to the rules of thermodynamics, just like any other closed system. Thermodynamic principles govern cellular functions including metabolism and energy transport. Biological systems' structure and behaviour can also be understood in light of these rules.

Thermodynamics is important in environmental research and climate modelling because it elucidates the pathways by which energy moves through Earth's ecosystems and how greenhouse gases function.

Thermodynamics is also used in the study of phase transitions, the properties of materials at different temperatures and pressures, and the design of innovative materials with desired characteristics in the field of material science (number six on the list).

The laws of thermodynamics are used in the study of astrophysics and cosmology to learn about the behaviour of heavenly bodies, the birth of stars and galaxies, and the ultimate fate of the universe. Implications for Future ResearchEven though the rules of thermodynamics give a solid foundation for studying energy and matter, scientists are still looking for exceptions in more complicated systems and more extreme settings. For instance:

1. Nanoscale and Quantum Thermodynamics: Scientists are looking into the application of thermodynamics to nanoscale systems and quantum mechanical phenomena, both of which may behave differently than expected by classical thermodynamics.

Non-equilibrium and emergent behaviours are commonplace in complex systems, such as biological systems and ecological networks, and thermodynamics is being applied to these areas.

Third, High-Energy Physics investigates thermodynamics in the setting of severe conditions, such as those created by particle collisions at the Large Hadron Collider (LHC).

4. Theoretical Extensions: To characterise systems outside of equilibrium, scientists are proposing theoretical extensions of thermodynamics such as non-equilibrium thermodynamics.

The Principles That Hold All Forms of Matter and Energy Together
There are few more fundamental or unifying principles in science than the rules of thermodynamics. They control the properties of energy and matter on sizes ranging from the microscopic to the macroscopic. from subatomic particles to the vastness of the cosmos. Our knowledge of the physical world, technological progress, and the pursuit of new knowledge are all underpinned by these rules.

The laws of thermodynamics are a cornerstone of scientific inquiry and a tribute to the power of human understanding in fields as iverse as the construction of energy-efficient motors, the understanding of biological interactions, the research of climate change, and the ration of the cosmos. They help us understand the underlying structure of the cosmos and equip us to navigate it and control its elements of energy and matter.

7.2 Enthalpy, Entropy, and Gibbs Free Energy

What Drives Chemical Reactions? An Exploration of Enthalpy, Entropy, and Gibbs Free Energy

Enthalpy, entropy, and Gibbs free energy are key concepts in chemistry and thermodynamics that help scientists make sense of chemical reactions and physical processes. These basic thermodynamic parameters shed light on the reversibility, reversal potential, and energy changes that accompany reactions. All the way from chemistry and physics to biology and environmental science are affected by the concepts of enthalpy, entropy, and Gibbs free energy, which we will examine in detail below.

Enthalpy: Getting to the Heart of the Matter

In thermodynamics, the enthalpy (H) of a system at a given pressure is a measure of its total heat content. Both the system's own potential energy and the energy of its surroundings (usually in the form of pressure-volume work) are factored in. The field of chemistry relies heavily on calculations of enthalpy to understand chemical processes and phase transitions.

The enthalpy change (denoted by the symbol "H") is a key thermodynamic variable in chemical reactions. A positive value indicates that heat is being absorbed by the process, whereas a negative value indicates that heat is being released. Standard enthalpy change (H°) is the enthalpy change of a reaction measured under standard conditions.

There are a number of important uses for enthalpy:

The enthalpy change (H) is a measure of the amount of heat added or removed from a system during a chemical process. It's a must-know for figuring out the temperature changes that accompany processes like combustion and phase changes.

Second, according to Hess's Law, the enthalpy change of a reaction is the same regardless of which pathway it takes. With this technique, researchers can determine a reaction's H by adding up the changes in enthalpy caused by a chain of similar reactions.

Calorimetry, the study of heat variations, is the third branch of science in this list. Calorimetry relies heavily on the idea of enthalpy in order to calculate the energy changes that occur during various processes, such as bomb calorimetry for combustion reactions.

Entropy — The Degree of Disorganisation

The degree of disorder or unpredictability in a system is denoted by the entropy symbol, S. Thermodynamics and statistical mechanics rely heavily on this idea. The direction and spontaneity of physical and chemical processes can be gleaned from the value of entropy.

As stated by the second law of thermodynamics, there is an inherent tendency for systems to evolve towards states of increased entropy over time. Naturally, processes that increase entropy are more likely to occur, whereas those that lower it are suppressed.

The concept of entropy is useful in many contexts:

Chemical Reactions: The change in entropy, S, helps establish whether a reaction is spontaneous or not in chemical reactions. An increase in S indicates a propensity towards spontaneity due to an increase in disorder, whereas a decrease in S indicates a lack of spontaneity.

In statistical mechanics, entropy is proportional to the number of possible microstates (different ways) of realising a macrostate (observable state). It connects the tiny world of particles with the larger characteristics of matter.

Entropy is strongly linked to the ideas of heat transport and heat engines, which brings us to our third topic: Thermal Processes. Changes in entropy, for instance, are crucial to the performance of heat engines like steam turbines and internal combustion engines.

The Reaction Engine That Is Gibbs Free Energy

As a thermodynamic property, Gibbs free energy (abbreviated G) integrates the ideas of enthalpy and entropy. An essential indicator of whether or not a certain chemical or physical process would occur spontaneously under test conditions.

A major sign of spontaneity is the shift in Gibbs free energy, denoted by the symbol "G."

For a process to be considered spontaneous under the specified conditions, the Gibbs free energy (G) must be negative. There will be a gradual return to equilibrium.

An increase in the Gibbs free energy, G, above zero indicates that the process being studied is not spontaneous under the parameters under consideration.

When G is zero, there is no net change in the system and the process has reached equilibrium.

In the following equation, G = H + S, where H and S are the enthalpy and entropy changes, respectively.

$\Delta G = \Delta H - T\Delta S$

Where H is the enthalpy change.

- S represents the entropy transition.
T is the Kelvin scale of absolute temperature.

In a variety of contexts, Gibbs free energy is useful:

First, in the realm of chemical reactions, G can be used to ascertain whether or not a certain reaction is spontaneous under study. It's all-encompassing evaluation of spontaneity takes into account both the heat energy change (H) and the entropy change (S).

2. Phase changes: G aids in predicting the conditions under which phase changes take place, such as the melting of ice or the evaporation of a liquid. It is common practise to use G when creating phase diagrams.

The third application of G is in the study of chemical equilibrium. When the reaction rates in both directions are equal, as they are at equilibrium, $G = 0$.

For the study of biological reactions, enzyme catalysis, and cellular activities, the concept of Gibbs free energy is crucial. It aids in determining the likelihood that a response will take place within a living creature.

Importance and Practical Applications

Understanding and foreseeing a vast array of natural and anthropogenic processes requires an intimate familiarity with enthalpy, entropy, and Gibbs free energy:

These thermodynamic characteristics are critical for maximising the efficiency of chemical processes, including those used to make medicines, fuels, and fertilisers. They are used by chemists and engineers to plan out optimal reaction routes and regulate experimental settings.

In the field of environmental science, knowing the thermodynamics of chemical reactions is crucial for determining the effects of pollution, how greenhouse gases behave, and where harmful substances end up after being released into the environment.

BIOCHEMISTRY AND PHYSIOLOGY, PART 3 Biochemical reactions, enzyme activity, and cellular activities are all under the control of these thermodynamic parameters of biological systems. Our knowledge of metabolism and energy transmission in biological systems is grounded in the principles of thermodynamics.

Four Conversion Parameters for Energy: Enthalpy and Gibbs

power plants, engines, and fuel cells, to name a few, rely heavily on the principles of free energy for their design and operation. When it comes to creating renewable energy sources, thermodynamics is crucial.

In the study of phase changes, material properties, and the creation of new materials with desirable qualities, thermodynamics plays a crucial role.

Implications for Future Research

While enthalpy, entropy, and the Gibbs free energy are all well-established concepts, their applications to non-equilibrium processes and systems, such as biological macromolecules and nanoscale materials, are still the subject of active investigation. Scientists are interested in learning more about these thermodynamic properties under unusual and extreme situations.

New materials can be designed and chemical processes can be optimised because to improvements in computational chemistry and molecular modelling that have allowed scientists to more accurately predict thermodynamic properties.

The Forces That Drive Chemistry and Beyond

The behaviour of matter and energy in the cosmos is governed by the laws of enthalpy, entropy, and Gibbs free energy. These universal principles shed light on the nature, course, and energy of chemical, physical, and biological processes. They are necessary for comprehending the mechanisms behind reactions, the stabilisation of systems, and the transformation of energy.

Enthalpy, entropy, and Gibbs free energy are at the core of scientific innovation and discovery across a wide range of fields, including the design of ecologically friendly chemical processes, the creation of innovative materials, and the search for sustainable energy solutions. Their utility extends to many fields, influencing how we view the natural world and paving the way for further scientific discovery and technological development in the future.

Chapter 8:
Synthetic Organic Chemistry

8.1 Introduction to Organic Compounds

An Overview of Organic Chemistry: The Basic Chemicals of Life

The building blocks of all known life are organic molecules. All living things have these carbon-based compounds as their foundation, and they are also crucial to countless chemical reactions that build our world. In this investigation, we will look into the nature of organic compounds, including their basic properties, the variety of carbon-containing molecules, their importance in biology and chemistry, and their many scientific uses.

The carbon atom is the organic world's structural lynchpin.

Carbon, a unique and adaptable element, is central to organic chemistry. The extraordinary variety of compounds that can be created is due to carbon's capacity to make stable covalent bonds with other atoms, including itself. Because of this quality, carbon may build the structural framework for an infinite number of chemical compounds, making up the backbone of organic molecules.

Long chains, branching structures, and intricate three-dimensional arrangements are all possible because to the bonding capabilities of carbon atoms. There is an incredible diversity of organic molecules because carbon may create single, double, or triple bonds with other elements including hydrogen, oxygen, nitrogen, and sulphur.

Important Traits of Organic Substances

Several distinguishing features set organic substances apart from their inorganic counterparts:

Carbon-hydrogen (C-H) bonds are the most common type of bond in organic molecules. These bonds are characteristic of many organic compounds but are not exclusive to organic chemistry.

2. Complex Molecular Structures: The molecules of organic compounds might be as simple as hydrocarbons or as complex as proteins and nucleic acids.

Third, Covalent Bonding, in which electrons are shared between atoms, is characteristic of most organic molecules. The stability of organic compounds depends on this kind of electron transfer.

Carbon skeletons or backbones are common in organic molecules and provide the molecular framework. Carbon atoms in these skeletons are arranged in a wide variety of ways.

The Richness and Variety of Organic Substances

There is a wide variety of molecules that make up organic compounds, all of which have certain roles to play. These are some of the most important groups of organic compounds:

Hydrocarbons are a class of organic molecules that consist of only carbon and hydrogen. Saturated hydrocarbons (alkanes), unsaturated hydrocarbons (alkenes), and unsaturated hydrocarbons (alkynes) are the three primary categories. Hydrocarbons can be found in a wide variety of organic materials, including fossil fuels, natural gas, and natural oils.

Alcohols, which can have anywhere from one to four hydroxyl (-OH) groups, are another type of organic molecule. One common example is ethanol, the alcohol found in many popular drinks.
Carboxylic acids, which are common in organic acids, have a carboxyl group (-COOH) in their chemical structure. Vinegar contains the carboxylic acid acetic acid.

Inorganic substances with one or more amino groups (-NH2) are called amines, the fourth class of organic molecules. The amino acids used to construct proteins are itself an amine.

In the presence of an alcohol, a carboxylic acid can react to produce an ester. They can be found in a wide variety of natural perfumes and flavours, and frequently have a sweet, fruity aroma.

Ketones and aldehydes are defined by the presence of a carbonyl group (C=O) in their chemical structure (see number 6). Solvent acetone is an aldehyde, and the more well-known aldehyde formaldehyde is an example of a ketone.

Polymers are big molecules that consist of monomer units linked together in a chain. Natural polymers like DNA, proteins, and cellulose, and manufactured polymers like plastics, are all included.

Importance of Organic Substances in Living Systems.

Organic substances are fundamental to the functioning of all known forms of life. In biology, there are four major groups of organic compounds:

Carbon, hydrogen, and oxygen atoms make up the organic molecules known as carbohydrates. They are essential for life because they provide a means of obtaining energy. Glucose, starch, and cellulose are a few examples.

Lipids, which include fats, oils, and phospholipids, are a broad class of chemical molecules. They are essential for storing energy, forming the structure of cell membranes, and transmitting signals. Lipids play a role in long-term energy storage and are crucial to the proper functioning of cell membranes.

Proteins, which are made up of amino acids, are enormous, complicated chemical molecules. Enzymes catalyse biochemical reactions, provide structural support, and transport molecules within cells, among many other roles they play in living creatures.

Nucleic acids, such as DNA and RNA, are molecules that can store and pass on genetic information. They play a crucial role in the processes of DNA replication and gene expression in all known forms of life.

Organic compounds' Rapidly Expanding Scientific Applications

Beyond biology, many other scientific fields and economic sectors make use of knowledge of organic substances.

One branch of chemistry, known as "organic chemistry," investigates the creation, structure, and reactions of organic substances. It plays a crucial role in advancing medicine, materials research, and industrial chemistry.

Organic chemicals constitute the backbone of the pharmaceutical industry and the search for new medicines. Medicinal chemists plan and create organic compounds with useful medicinal effects.

Organic compounds are employed in the production of many different types of materials in the field of Materials Science; they include plastics, fibres, and adhesives. Electronics and packaging, for example, have benefited greatly from developments in organic materials.

In the study of contaminants and their effects on ecosystems, organic molecules play an important role in environmental chemistry. Remediating polluted environments requires knowledge of organic contaminants and how they degrade.

5. Agriculture: Organic chemistry is utilised to improve crop yields and pest control through the creation of insecticides, fertilisers, and herbicides.

Implications for Future Research

The discipline of organic chemistry is one that is constantly expanding and developing.

First, Synthetic Chemistry: New methods for the synthesis of organic substances are continually being developed, allowing for the development of cutting-edge materials and medicines.

Second, "Sustainable Chemistry," or "Green Chemistry," seeks to lessen the negative effects of the chemical industry on the environment through the creation of greener methods for producing and using organic molecules.

Medicinal Chemistry (3): New medications and cures for a variety of ailments, including as cancer, infectious diseases, and neurological disorders, are being discovered thanks to advancements in medicinal chemistry.

Nanotechnology, number four: organic molecules are utilised to create nanomaterials and nanoscale devices with potential uses in electronics, sensing, and medicine.

The Foundations of Life and Science, Final Thoughts

Organic chemicals form the basis of all life on Earth and have inspired many scientific and technological advancements. Organic compounds are the fundamental elements of life and the key to understanding the mysteries of the natural world, and they range in size from the tiny molecules that power cellular functions to the complex polymers that form the basis of materials science.

Our knowledge of these molecules and their uses in various sectors grow as organic chemistry research progresses. Organic compounds continue to be at the vanguard of scientific inquiry and human progress, moulding the world we live in and the future we may imagine through their use in the manufacturing of life-saving pharmaceuticals, the design of sustainable materials, and the discovery of new frontiers in nanotechnology.

8.2 Hydrocarbons: Alkanes, Alkenes, Alkynes

The building blocks of organic chemistry are hydrocarbons such as alkanes, alkenes, and alkynes.

Hydrocarbons make up the bare bones of organic chemistry as the most elementary of all organic substances. Hydrocarbons, which consist of only carbon and hydrogen atoms, display amazing structural and property diversity. The three primary categories of hydrocarbons are the alkanes, alkenes, and alkynes, each of which has its own unique bonding patterns and properties. In this examination of hydrocarbons, we will look into the distinctions between alkanes, alkenes, and alkynes; their role in organic chemistry; their practical uses; and the far-reaching effects they have on academia, business, and government.

Saturated hydrocarbons (or alkanes)

The simplest class of hydrocarbons, alkanes feature just single bonds between carbon atoms and hydrogen atoms. They are called "saturated" hydrocarbons because their carbon skeletons are completely filled with hydrogen atoms.

Principal Alkane Characteristics:

One distinguishing feature of alkanes is the occurrence of single covalent connections between carbon atoms (hence the name "alkane"). These single bonds permit rotation about the carbon-carbon axis, making the final structure quite malleable.

The tetrahedral geometry of alkanes is the result of the formation of four sigma () bonds between each carbon atom. This tetrahedral arrangement produces a symmetrical three-dimensional structure by optimising the bond angles.

Thirdly, alkanes are considered "saturated" because adding more hydrogen atoms would disrupt the carbon-carbon bonds and render the molecule unstable. They are distinguished from unsaturated hydrocarbons such as alkenes and alkynes by this feature.

Four, their General Formula is C_nH_{2n+2}, where "n" is the number of carbon atoms in the alkane. The formula shows how the number of carbon atoms in an alkane correlates with the number of hydrogen atoms.

5. Hydrophobic: Alkanes, like other hydrocarbons, are normally insoluble in water but soluble in nonpolar solvents.

The Importance of Alkanes

There are several uses and industries where alkanes are indispensable:

First, there are fossil fuels; the majority of the hydrocarbons in petroleum are alkanes. Petrol, diesel fuel and natural gas are three of the world's most important energy sources made possible by the petroleum industry.

Alkanes are used as precursors in the chemical industry for the production of a wide range of organic chemicals. They serve as raw materials in the chemical industry, where they are transformed into things like polymers and solvents.

Thirdly, alkane combustion is a major contributor to climate change due to the release of carbon dioxide (CO_2). Cleaner alternatives to alkane-based fuels are the focus of scientific research and commercial innovation.

Those unsaturated hydrocarbons are called alkenes.

There is at least one carbon-carbon double bond (C=C) in the hydrocarbons known as alkenes. This unsaturation is brought about by the presence of a double bond, which can undergo further chemical processes to produce more bonds.

Important Aspects of Alkenes:

First and foremost, alkenes have a sigma ( ) and pi ( ) double bond between their carbon atoms. Because the pi bond prevents rotation around the carbon-carbon axis, the molecule is locked into a specific shape.

In some alkenes, the arrangement of the substituent groups around the double bond can be either cis (on the same side) or trans (on opposing sides), a phenomenon known as cis-trans isomerism. The result of this isomerism is a variety of novel chemical and physical characteristics.

Third, alkenes can be converted to alkanes through a process called hydrogenation, in which hydrogen atoms are added across the double bond. This reaction is commonly employed in the food sector to convert liquid vegetable oils into solid fats.

4 General Formula: The general formula for alkenes is C_nH_{2n}, where "n" denotes the number of carbon atoms in the alkene. The presence of double bonds in this formula indicates a lower hydrogen content than in alkanes.

Importance of Alkenes

In a number of contexts, alkenes are indispensable:

Alkenes are used in the production of polymers including polyethylene, polypropylene, and polyvinyl chloride (PVC), which have many applications in industry and consumer goods.

Chemical processes: Alkenes participate in a wide variety of chemical processes, including addition reactions, in which new atoms or groups are added to the double bond. The synthesis of many different types of organic molecules relies on these processes.

Alkenes are found in compounds with biological significance, like fatty acids and terpenes, according to biochemistry. They have an important role in biomolecule structure and function.

Triple-bonded hydrocarbons (or alkynes)

One characteristic of alkynes, a type of hydrocarbon, is the existence of a carbon-carbon triple bond (CC). The molecular structure is made extremely stiff and unsaturated by the presence of this triple bond.

Important Traits of Alkynes

To begin, Triple Bonds are present in Alkynes.

 triple bond between carbon atoms, consisting of a sigma () bond and two pi () bonds, as a minimum. Molecular geometry is linear because the triple bond prevents rotation about the carbon-carbon axis.

In alkynes, the hydrogen is bonded to a carbon atom that is close to the triple bond, making the molecule acidic. Alkynyl anions can be formed when this hydrogen undergoes processes like deprotonation.

Number of carbon atoms in the alkyne is the "n" in the generic formula for alkynes, which is C_nH_{2n-2}. The presence of triple bonds is reflected in this formula, which indicates a lower hydrogen content than alkanes.

The Importance of Alkynes

There are a number of crucial uses for alkynes:

In organic synthesis, alkynes are useful for building complex compounds and creating carbon-carbon bonds via reactions such as the Sonogashira coupling.

To make specific polymers and conductive materials, for example, some alkynes and their derivatives are used in materials science.

In analytical chemistry and biochemistry, alkynes are employed as chemical probes and reagents for the detection and labelling of particular functional groups.

Impact and Real-World Applications

The hydrocarbons, which include alkanes, alkenes, and alkynes, have far-reaching effects on manufacturing, power generation, and daily living.

Alkanes are a key ingredient of petrol and diesel fuel, which are used to power cars, trucks and other vehicles.

Alkenes are the building blocks of polymer synthesis, which in turn has led to the development of numerous materials used in the manufacture of containers, building supplies, and consumer items.

Hydrocarbons, in the form of fossil fuels, are a significant contributor to the production of energy. Methane (an alkane) is the primary component of natural gas, which has many use in the heating, electricity generating, and manufacturing sectors.

Hydrocarbons are a vital raw element for the chemical industry, which manufactures everything from drugs to cleaning supplies to fertiliser.Hydrocarbon combustion results in increased air pollution and greenhouse gas emissions, which brings us to our fifth and last environmental consideration. Cleaner energy alternatives are being developed and the environmental impact of hydrocarbon consumption is being mitigated by continual efforts.

Implications for Future Research

Hydrocarbons research keeps moving forward, tackling new problems and opening up exciting avenues.

1. Green Chemistry: Researchers are working to find more efficient and less wasteful ways to produce and use hydrocarbons in everyday life.

2. Alternative Energy: Efforts are being made to discover low-carbon energy and fuel sources other than fossil fuels. Examples of this include biofuels and hydrogen.

Thirdly, Materials Science: New discoveries in this area are paving the way for novel uses of hydrocarbons in industries like nanotechnology, flexible electronics, and renewable energy.

4. Catalysis: Studies in catalysis attempt to boost the efficiency of chemical reactions using hydrocarbons, hence decreasing the energy required and negative effects on the environment.Hydrocarbons, a Versatile World of their OwnHydrocarbons, such as alkanes, alkenes, and alkynes, form the backbone of organic chemistry and find widespread use in a variety of fields, such as manufacturing, energy generation, and materials science. They are crucial in the production of a wide variety of organic chemicals and materials due to their versatile architectures and high reactivity. The environmental risks associated with their widespread application highlight the need for new knowledge and methods to safely and responsibly unlock the potential of hydrocarbons. As our knowledge of these substances grows, so will their influence on the future of business, technology, and our approach to energy and building materials.

Chapter 9:
A Brief Introduction to Inorganic Chemistry

9.1 Properties of Inorganic Compounds

Non-organic chemistry and its wide variety of useful properties.

The wide and varied group of chemical molecules known as inorganic compounds plays an essential role in chemistry, materials science, and technology. Inorganic compounds, in contrast to organic compounds based on carbon-hydrogen (C-H) bonds, are largely formed of elements other than carbon and include a vast variety of substances with unique properties and uses. In this investigation of inorganic compounds, we will examine their essential features, physical and chemical properties, scientific importance, and industrial applications.

Important Features of Inorganic Substances:

First and foremost, inorganic compounds are distinguished by the fact that they do not have carbon-hydrogen (C-H) bonds. Metals, nonmetals, and metalloids make up the bulk of their make-up instead.

Two types of bonding seen in inorganic materials are ionic and covalent. Electrostatic forces hold ions together in ionic compounds, which are formed when electrons are transferred from one atom to another. However, in covalent compounds, electrons are transferred between atoms.

Sodium chloride is a simple binary molecule, but inorganic compounds also include more complex coordination compounds like metal complexes and mineral compounds like quartz, all of which have their own unique chemical compositions.

Fourth, many inorganic chemicals can be dissolved in water and, because of the presence of ions, can conduct electricity. This quality is essential for a wide range of uses, including as battery electrolytes and electronic conductors.

Inorganic compounds' physical characteristics:

There is a wide variation in the melting and boiling temperatures of inorganic compounds due to factors including ionic or covalent interaction, molecule size, and crystal structure. Strong electrostatic interactions between ions, for instance, cause melting and boiling temperatures in ionic compounds to be relatively high.

2. Density: The density of inorganic compounds can range from very low (for example, aluminium) to very high (for example, lead).

3. Colour: Inorganic compounds can display a wide colour palette, typically attributable to the presence of metal ions or transition metal complexes that absorb particular colours of light. Pigments and dyes rely on this quality greatly.

Fourth, many inorganic substances are electrically conductive when dissolved in water or molten. When ionic materials are broken down into their component ions, electricity can flow through them.

Chemical characteristics of inorganic substances:

Inorganic substances, notably metals, are able to undergo a wide variety of chemical reactions, resulting in oxides, sulphides, and other compounds.

Acid-Base Behaviour: Inorganic substances can be either acidic or basic. Oxides of metals, for instance, can interact with water to generate hydroxides, demonstrating basic behaviour, while oxides of other elements can do the opposite, producing acids.

Redox (oxidation-reduction) reactions involve a wide variety of inorganic substances. Redox processes can cause corrosion in metals, for instance.

Importance in the Natural Sciences:

There are far-reaching consequences for inorganic substances in several scientific fields:

1. In the field of chemical, the study of inorganic substances and their synthesis, characterisation, and reactivity is known as inorganic chemistry. This discipline is crucial for learning about the characteristics and actions of atoms and molecules.

Inorganic compounds are essential to the field of materials science, where they are utilised to create electrical components, building materials, and even aeronautical components like ceramics, semiconductors, and superconductors.

Third, Geology: Geologists may learn a great deal about Earth's composition, geological processes, and the development of important resources like ores through the study of minerals and mineral compounds.

Coordination Chemistry, which studies the characteristics and behaviour of metal complexes with ligands, relies heavily on coordination compounds, a subset of inorganic chemicals.

5Environmental research: Inorganic compounds have an important role in pollution, water chemistry, and the behaviour of heavy metals in ecosystems, making them an important part of environmental research.

Inorganic Compounds in Everyday Life:

The range of fields that can benefit from inorganic chemicals is wide.

First, in metallurgy, inorganic compounds are crucial in metal extraction and refining. Iron is extracted from compounds such as iron ore (hematite).

2. Catalysis: Inorganic compounds are commonly used as catalysts in chemical reactions across a variety of contexts, including industrial operations, automotive catalytic converters, and the synthesis of chemicals and pharmaceuticals.

To make transistors, diodes, and integrated circuits, the electronics industry relies on semiconductors, which are inorganic substances like silicon and gallium arsenide.

4. Ceramics: Ceramics have uses in electronics, aerospace, and construction, and are made from inorganic compounds like alumina (aluminium oxide) and zirconia (zirconium dioxide).

Drugs: Antacids, dental fillings, and contrast agents for x-rays are just a few examples of how inorganic compounds find their way into pharmaceuticals.

Construction uses inorganic compounds like cement and concrete because of their strength and longevity in the built environment.

7. Agriculture: Inorganic chemicals like fertilisers increase crop output and agricultural productivity by providing critical nutrients to plants.

Problems and Ongoing Studies:

1. Green Chemistry: The study of how to synthesise and use inorganic substances in ways that are less harmful to the environment and produce less waste.

Inorganic nanoparticles and nanomaterials are finding new and exciting uses in industries including health, electronics, and energy storage thanks to advancements in nanotechnology.

3. Materials Engineering: New inorganic materials with unique features, like superconductors, photovoltaic materials, and high-strength alloys, are the focus of ongoing research in materials engineering.

Inorganic chemicals and materials are being developed by scientists for use in environmental remediation, which includes cleaning polluted air and water and dealing with contaminated soil.

Inorganic Compounds: A Wide Variety with Many Applications

Inorganic compounds are a large and important class of chemicals with foundational roles in many fields of study and industries. Despite their absence of carbon-hydrogen bonds, inorganic compounds play an essential role in many scientific disciplines. These include chemistry, materials science, geology, and even environmental studies. Inorganic compounds have a wide range of practical uses, from metallurgy and electronics to building and agriculture, which have shaped industries and enhanced the quality of life. The potential of inorganic compounds is still being explored, leading to new solutions to environmental problems, technological breakthroughs, and scientific advancements.

9.2 Transition Metals and Coordination Compounds

The Diverse World of Metal Complexes: Transition Metals and Coordination Compounds

The transition metals are an essential part of the periodic table due to their prominence and the wide range of applications for their chemistry. Coordination compounds, also called metal complexes, are unique to transition metals including iron, copper, and platinum. The fascinating intricacy of coordination compounds and the crucial functions they play in many scientific and practical contexts make them fascinating subjects. Through this investigation of coordination compounds and transition metals, we will learn about the unique properties of transition metals, the fundamentals of coordination chemistry, and the far-reaching impact of metal complexes in disciplines like biology, catalysis, and materials science.

The Transition Metals Are Extremely Diverse Chemically

In the periodic table, transition metals are located in the centre block, from groups 3 to 12. Their exceptional qualities, which include:

1. Variable Oxidation States: Transition metals are able to rapidly receive or lose electrons in chemical processes due to their ability to exist in a number of oxidation states. This allows them to build compounds with a wide variety of other elements.

Transition metals can form coordination complexes with a wide variety of coordination numbers and geometries, which is referred to as "coordination diversity." Octahedral, tetrahedral, and square-planar geometries are all rather common.

3. Coloured Compounds: Electronic transitions within the d orbitals of the metal ion give many transition metal compounds their vivid

colours. The brilliant hues of transition metal complexes can be traced back to this characteristic.

In the fields of materials science and magnetism, compounds containing transition metals that display magnetic behaviour are of great interest.

Coordinated chemistry, or the study of metal complexes,

The study of coordination compounds, which have a metal atom or ion covalently bound to surrounding molecules or ions called ligands, is the subject of coordination chemistry. There are a few fundamental rules in coordination chemistry:

One's coordination number indicates how many bonds there are between the metal centre and the ligands. The geometry of the coordination complex is set by this factor.

Two, Ligands are molecules or ions that form coordination bonds with the metal atom via donor atoms. Water (H_2O), ammonia (NH_3), and chloride (Cl) are all examples of common ligands.

Chelation (3): This process takes place when a ligand makes numerous bonds with the centre metal atom, resulting in a ring-like shape. The complex is more stable after being chelated.

4. Isomerism: Geometric (cis-trans) and structural (linkage) isomerism are two types of isomerism that can be seen in coordination complexes.

Coordination compounds are important in many ways.

The significance of coordination chemicals extends to many different scientific fields.

1. Biology: Metal complexes serve as cofactors in enzymes and participate in critical activities including oxygen transport (haemoglobin) and photosynthesis (chlorophyll) in biological systems.

To make chemicals, medicines, and polymers, transition metal complexes serve as catalysts in numerous industrial processes. Catalysts based on platinum can be found in fuel cells and organic synthesis uses Wilkinson's catalyst.

Third, in the field of Materials Science, coordination compounds are important for the creation of new technologies including superconductors, photovoltaics, and luminous materials for use in electronics and lighting.

4. Medicine: Metal-based chemotherapy medicines like cisplatin were developed because some metal complexes show interesting anticancer qualities.

5. Environmental Science: The role of coordination compounds in environmental processes such as the fate of heavy metals in ecosystems and wastewater treatment is investigated.

Coordination Compounds in the Real World:

In many fields, coordination molecules have found useful applications:

The manufacturing of plastics, fine chemicals, and pharmaceuticals all use transition metal complexes as catalysts in industrial operations.Coordination compounds are used to make conductive materials and luminous displays, both of which find widespread application in electronics manufacturing.

Thirdly, platinum-based coordination complexes are frequently utilised in chemotherapy for the treatment of cancer.

The removal of heavy metals and other pollutants from the environment is accomplished by using metal complexes in wastewater treatment (see also: Environmental Remediation).

Photovoltaics, the development of solar cells and photovoltaic materials, utilises certain metal complexes for the production of renewable energy.Problems and Ongoing Studies:Challenges and opportunities in coordination chemistry research continue to be investigated.

First, "Green Chemistry" is an effort to find less wasteful and more energy-efficient ways to create and utilise metal complexes in veryday applications.Researchers in the field of Bioinorganic Chemistry study the function of metal complexes in living organisms and work to make safer, more effective metal-based pharmaceuticals.

The development of more effective and selective metal catalysts for a wide range of chemical processes constitutes an area of advancement known as catalysis.

4. Materials Science: New metal complexes with interesting electrical, magnetic, and optical properties are being investigated for use in high-tech materials.Metal Complexes: A Wide-Ranging Family of Materials

The study and development of new technologies often begins with studies of transition metals and coordination molecules. These adaptable elements and the complexes they form are crucial to deciphering the microscopic and macroscopic properties of matter. Coordination compounds serve crucial roles in the critical processes of biology, the catalysis of industrial operations, and the development of new materials and technology. Our capacity to use the amazing features of metal complexes for the betterment of society and the environment will grow as coordination chemistry research advances.

Chapter 10:
Laboratory Methods and Analytical Chemistry

10.1 Techniques for Chemical Analysis

Chemical Analysis Methods: A Key to the Universe

Chemical analysis is fundamental to modern research because it reveals the molecular and atomic levels of matter's composition, structure, and behaviour. Many different methods have been devised to investigate the chemical world, from determining what elements are present in a complex combination to learning how substances behave throughout a reaction. In this review of chemical analysis methods, we will examine some of the most basic and cutting-edge approaches, as well as their underlying concepts, practical applications, and central role in a wide range of scientific fields.

The First Peer into the Spectrum, or Spectroscopy

The production of a spectrum through the interaction of matter with electromagnetic radiation like light is the basis of the strong analytical tool known as spectroscopy. This spectrum can tell us a lot about the chemical make-up and molecular structure of a material. Methods central to spectroscopy include:

The absorption of both ultraviolet (UV) and visible light by molecules can be measured by UV-Vis spectroscopy, yielding information about electronic transitions. Chemistry and biology rely on it to determine the relative concentration of compounds.

Absorption of infrared radiation can be measured with IR spectroscopy to gain insight into the vibrational and rotational modes of chemical bonds. It is helpful for determining which parts of organic compounds serve as functional groups.

- NMR Spectroscopy (Nuclear Magnetic Resonance): Magnetic and radiofrequency radiation interact with atomic nuclei in nuclear magnetic resonance spectroscopy. In chemistry and biochemistry, it is commonly employed for the analysis of chemical molecules, the research of protein structures, and the study of reaction mechanisms.

- Mass Spectrometry (MS): By analysing the mass-to-charge ratio of ions, mass spectrometry can reveal details about a compound's molecular weight and chemical make-up. It plays a crucial role in identifying organic molecules and in the fields of proteomics and metabolomics.

Chromatography, the Art of Disentangling Complex Substances:

Chromatography refers to a group of separation methods in which components of a mixture are separated and analysed based on their relative affinities for a stationary phase and a mobile phase. Techniques used frequently in chromatography include:

Gas chromatography (GC) is a technique for separating volatile substances in a gaseous mobile phase, making it useful for the analysis of organic molecules such as hydrocarbons, insecticides, and medicines.

To separate a wide variety of chemicals, such as pharmaceuticals, biomolecules, and environmental toxins, one can use liquid chromatography (LC), which uses a liquid mobile phase.

The use of high-pressure pumps in HPLC allows for quicker separations and improved resolution, making it an ideal technique for analysing complicated mixtures.

The stationary phase in thin-layer chromatography (TLC) is deposited in a very thin layer on a solid substrate. It has many applications, including the rapid qualitative interpretation of data and the observation of chemical processes.

Weighting Molecules using Mass Spectrometry (MS)

The analytical method known as mass spectrometry can be used to learn about a molecule's mass, content, and structure. It has many applications and is commonly used:

Proteins, peptides, and nucleic acids can all be analysed using Electrospray Ionisation (ESI) MS. Since it uses a solution to produce ions, it works well with big, polar compounds.

Matrix-assisted laser desorption/ionization mass spectrometry (MALDI MS) In the fields of proteomics and lipidomics, MALDI MS is utilised to examine big macromolecules. Laser light is used to irradiate a sample, producing ions.

- Tandem Mass Spectrometry (MS/MS): MS/MS consists of two steps of mass analysis, which enables the identification of individual fragments and elucidates the structure of complicated molecules.

Molecular Structures Revealed by X-ray Crystallography 4

Small chemical molecules, proteins, and inorganic compounds can all be analysed using X-ray crystallography to reveal their three-dimensional structures. The X-rays are scattered by the crystal lattice, creating a diffraction pattern that can be analysed statistically to reveal the atomic structure.

By elucidating the three-dimensional structures of proteins, enzymes, and other biomolecules, the field of structural biology has been revolutionised by the technique of Protein Crystallography. It can affect how we think about drugs and how we interpret biological processes.

X-ray crystallography can also be used to determine the structures of small molecules, both organic and inorganic, shedding light on their bonding patterns and three-dimensional atomic arrangement.

NMR Spectroscopy for Investigating Molecular Structure, Method 5

Nuclear magnetic resonance (NMR) spectroscopy is a flexible method for investigating molecules and their interactions. The magnetic characteristics of specific atomic nuclei, such as hydrogen (1H) and carbon-13 (13C), form the basis of this theory.

The use of 1H NMR for determining the 3D structure of organic compounds is widespread. Hydrogen atom counts and chemical conditions in various surroundings are revealed.

Two-dimensional nuclear magnetic resonance (NMR) spectroscopy includes methods like correlation spectroscopy (COSY) and heteronuclear single-quantum coherence (HSQC).

), reveal how the atoms in a molecule are connected to one another and how they interact with one another.

Solid-state nuclear magnetic resonance (NMR) is used to learn about the three-dimensional structure and dynamic behaviour of solid materials such catalysts, polymers, and biomolecules.

Understanding Electron Transfer (6. Electrochemistry)

Electrochemical methods are essential in electrochemistry, materials science, and environmental research because they are used to examine the flow of electrons in chemical reactions.

- Cyclic Voltammetry: In cyclic voltammetry, the voltage at an electrode is swept as the current is measured. It is employed in the analysis of electrochemical properties and the investigation of redox processes.

Electrochemical processes can be precisely regulated with the help of equipment called potentiostats and galvanostats, respectively.

Electrochemical impedance spectroscopy (EIS) is a technique that measures the impedance of an electrochemical system as a function of frequency to learn more about the kinetics of a reaction and the characteristics of the electrodes.

Thermal Analysis: Looking into Thermal Characteristics is the seventh method.

Methods of thermal analysis entail determining how changes in temperature or time affect the physical and chemical properties of substances. Techniques used frequently in thermal analysis include:

Differential Scanning Calorimetry (DSC) is a technique used to learn about the properties of a material by measuring the heat flow associated with phase transitions like melting and crystallisation.

Mass changes as a function of temperature or time are measured using thermogravimetric analysis (TGA), which can be used to learn about a material's make-up, breakdown, and stability.

Differential thermal analysis (DTA) is a technique that compares the variations in temperature between a sample and a standard during a series of carefully regulated heating and cooling cycles.

Microscopy, or "Eye in the Sky"

Microscopy methods allow for the microscopic examination and characterisation of material. Important types of microscopy include:

Visible light is used to magnify and examine samples in optical microscopy. Fluorescence and confocal microscopy are two microscopy methods that increase contrast and reveal finer details in samples.

- Electron Microscopy: Electron microscopes provide greater resolution images by using electron beams rather than light. Scanning electron microscopy (SEM) and transmission electron microscopy (TEM) reveal intricate structural details.

Nanotechnology and materials research benefit greatly from the use of atomic force microscopy (AFM) since it allows for the visualisation and manipulation of sample surfaces at the atomic scale.

Chromatography for Classifying and Isolating Compounds:

Chromatography refers to a group of separation methods in which components of a mixture are separated and analysed based on their relative affinities for a stationary phase and a mobile phase. Techniques used frequently in chromatography include:

Gas chromatography (GC) is a technique for separating volatile substances in a gaseous mobile phase, making it useful for the analysis of organic molecules such as hydrocarbons, insecticides, and medicines.

To separate a wide variety of chemicals, such as pharmaceuticals, biomolecules, and environmental toxins, one can use liquid chromatography (LC), which uses a liquid mobile phase.

The use of high-pressure pumps in HPLC allows for quicker separations and improved resolution, making it an ideal technique for analysing complicated mixtures.
The stationary phase in thin-layer chromatography (TLC) is deposited in a very thin layer on a solid substrate. It has many applications,

including the rapid qualitative interpretation of data and the observation of chemical processes.

10 Microscopy: A Look at the Invisible

Microscopy methods allow for the microscopic examination and characterisation of material. Important types of microscopy include:

Visible light is used to magnify and examine samples in optical microscopy. Fluorescence and confocal microscopy are two microscopy methods that increase contrast and reveal finer details in samples.

- Electron Microscopy: Electron microscopes provide greater resolution images by using electron beams rather than light. Scanning electron microscopy (SEM) and transmission electron microscopy (TEM) reveal intricate structural details.

Nanotechnology and materials research benefit greatly from the use of atomic force microscopy (AFM) since it allows for the visualisation and manipulation of sample surfaces at the atomic scale.

Applications in a Variety of Scientific Fields:

The aforementioned methods can be used in many different scientific fields:

In order to characterise compounds, identify unknown molecules, and investigate reaction mechanisms, chemical analysis techniques are essential in the field of chemistry.

Spectroscopy, mass spectrometry, and nuclear magnetic resonance (NMR) are crucial tools for analysing biomolecules, determining protein structures, and performing metabolomics in the field of biology.

Third, Materials Science: X-ray crystallography, microscopy, and thermal analysis are all crucial to comprehending the properties and structures of materials.

In the field of Environmental Science, chromatography and mass spectrometry are employed for the purpose of identifying and quantifying contaminants in the environment.

5. Pharmaceuticals: Drug analysis and quality control are performed using high-performance liquid chromatography (HPLC) and mass spectrometry.

6. Geology: The study of the composition and structure of minerals by X-ray diffraction (XRD) and electron microscopy.

Problems and Ongoing Studies:

The field of chemical analysis is ever-evolving in response to new problems:

1. Nanotechnology: The development of analytical methods for characterising nanoscale materials and structures is being driven by advancements in nanotechnology.

In order to rapidly screen a large number of samples, analytical devices are incorporating automation and robotics to do high-throughput analysis.

Thirdly, Data Analysis involves improving the understanding of complex analytical data through the use of cutting-edge methods like machine learning and artificial intelligence.

In the fourth area, called "Environmental Monitoring," scientists are working to improve detection and response times for environmental toxins.

Finishing Up: Chemical Analysis' Scientific Toolkit:
The development of sophisticated methods for chemical analysis has been crucial to the advancement of science and technology because it has allowed us to gain unprecedented insight into the nature of matter's composition, structure, and behaviour. These methods have a wide range of scientific applications, from the discovery of new chemicals to the analysis of environmental pollutants and protein structures. The strength and adaptability of chemical analysis continue to reveal the mysteries of nature and propel scientific and technological advancement as technology and multidisciplinary study grow.

10.2 Spectroscopy and Chromatography

Chromatography and Spectroscopy: Shining a Light on the Chemical Cosmos

Analytical chemistry would be nothing without spectroscopy and chromatography, the two mainstay techniques that give researchers access to the instruments necessary to decipher the chemical world. These methods, which grew out of the natural inquisitiveness of early scientists and have been honed over ages, are now fundamental to our ability to comprehend the nature and behaviour of matter. Our investigation into spectroscopy and chromatography will delve deeply into their fundamentals, practical applications, and far-reaching impact across many scientific fields and economic sectors.

Looking at the Spectrum Through Spectroscopy

Spectroscopy is a diverse area of study that makes use of many different methods. Spectroscopy, at its core, is the study of the resulting spectrum from the interaction of matter with electromagnetic radiation like light. This spectrum, typically represented by a graph or plot, can tell you a lot about the make-up and structure of a substance. The following are examples of well-known spectroscopic techniques:

Absorption of both ultraviolet (UV) and visible light by molecules can be measured by UV-Visible Spectroscopy (UV-Vis). It is commonly used in chemistry, biology, and environmental research to analyse the concentration of chemicals and provides insights into electronic transitions inside molecules.

Absorption of infrared light (which corresponds to vibrational and rotational modes of chemical bonds) is measured in IR spectroscopy. This method is essential in organic chemistry for determining the identities of functional groups in compounds.

- NMR Spectroscopy (Nuclear Magnetic Resonance): Using a magnetic field and radio waves, NMR spectroscopy is a flexible method for studying atomic nuclei. It is widely used in organic chemistry, structural biology, and biochemistry, and in the research of reaction mechanisms.

We use MS to refer to mass spectrometry. The mass-to-charge ratio of ions created from a sample is analysed by means of mass spectrometry. In domains like proteomics, metabolomics, and organic molecule identification, it is crucial since it may reveal the molecular weight and composition of chemicals.

Spectroscopy Basics:

The interactions between matter and electromagnetic radiation form the basis of spectroscopy's guiding principles.

The first process, Absorption and Emission, occurs when molecules raise their energy level by absorbing electromagnetic radiation. In contrast, they radiate energy as they decay back to a lower energy state. These absorption and emission processes are used by spectroscopic methods to learn about the chemical and physical characteristics of substances.

Second, a substance's chemical structure can be inferred from the particular wavelengths or frequencies of radiation absorbed or emitted by it. Scientists are able to identify substances and learn about their molecular structures by analysing these wavelengths or frequencies.

Quantization of Energy, or the existence of discrete, well-defined energy levels within atoms and molecules. Spectroscopy provides researchers with an in-depth look at the electronic and vibrational states of matter by allowing them to investigate these levels and transitions.

Spectroscopy's Many Uses

Numerous fields and industries can benefit from spectroscopy's many uses:

First, in the fields of chemistry and biochemistry, spectroscopy plays a crucial role in clarifying the structures of organic and inorganic substances, investigating the kinetics of chemical reactions, and characterising biomolecules including proteins, nucleic acids, and lipids.

2. Pharmaceutics: Spectroscopy is employed in identifying and quantifying active pharmaceutical components, evaluating purity, and monitoring chemical reactions in medication development and quality control.

Thirdly, spectroscopic techniques are used in environmental science to analyse toxins in air, water, and soil, which aids in environmental monitoring and cleanup.

4. Materials Science: Spectroscopy is used to study materials' properties, such as those of semiconductors, superconductors, and polymers, which contributes to the creation of cutting-edge materials for many uses.

Astronomy is the fifth field where spectroscopy is used extensively. From stars and planets to galaxies and interstellar clouds, astronomers utilise spectroscopy to learn more about their composition and physical features.

Chromatography: The Art of Disentangling Messy Blends

Chromatography refers to a group of analytical methods used to isolate and study individual substances within a larger mixture. The term "chromatography" comes from the Greek words "chroma" (colour) and "grapho" (to write) because the practise was once used to isolate dyes from plants. Differential interactions between components of a mixture and two phases—a stationary phase and a mobile phase—form the basis of chromatographic techniques. Techniques used frequently in chromatography include:

Gas chromatography (GC) is a technique for separating chemicals that are easily vaporised by using a gaseous mobile phase. It is commonly used for the analysis of hydrocarbons, insecticides, and pharmaceuticals. The fields of environmental monitoring and forensic analysis rely heavily on GC as an analytical tool.

Liquid chromatography (LC) is a powerful technique for the separation of many different types of substances, including medicines, biomolecules, and environmental pollutants, thanks to its use of a liquid mobile phase. HPLC is a high-pressure modification of LC that allows for quicker separations and improved resolution.

The stationary phase in thin-layer chromatography (TLC) is deposited in a very thin layer on a solid substrate. It has many applications in the laboratory, including rapid qualitative analysis and the observation of chemical processes.

To analyse inorganic anions and cations in environmental samples, water quality testing, and food analysis, one can use Ion Chromatography (IC), which focuses on the separation of ions.

Chromatographic Principles:

Differential component distribution between the stationary and mobile phases is essential to the chromatographic separation process. Some fundamentals are:

First, there is partitioning, which is when components of a mixture separate into the stationary phase and the mobile phase according to their affinities. Concentrations that have a higher affinity for the stationary phase will progress more slowly through the column, while those with a higher affinity for the mobile phase will elute more quickly.

Second, the Retention Time of a component is the time it takes to elute from the chromatographic column. The retention times of various compounds vary, allowing for easy categorization.

3. Column Selectivity: Precise separation of target compounds is possible with careful manipulation of the stationary phase and mobile phase. The success of chromatographic separations is heavily dependent on the selectivity of the column used.

Chromatography's Practical Uses

Many scientific and industrial fields make use of chromatography:

Chromatography is used in the pharmaceutical industry for quality control, drug development, and analysis of active pharmaceutical components, guaranteeing the purity and potency of drugs.

Second, chromatography is used in the food and beverage industry to test for and identify pollutants, additives, and flavour components, all of which contribute to the product's overall quality and safety.

Environmental evaluation and regulation are aided by chromatography's ability to detect and quantify contaminants in air, water, and soil.

The chemical manufacturing sector makes use of chromatography for product development and quality control by purifying and analysing substances.

5. Forensic Science: Chromatography is crucial in forensic analysis, allowing for the identification of narcotics, poisons, and other chemicals during criminal investigations.

6. Research and creation: Chromatography's insights into reaction kinetics and product purity are invaluable in the creation of novel materials, catalysts, and medicinal molecules.

Problems and Ongoing Studies:

Spectroscopy and chromatography are constantly developing to meet new needs and broaden their applications.

1. Miniaturisation: Scientists are working on compact and portable spectrometers and chromatographs for use in real-time diagnostics and other point-of-care settings.

In order to rapidly screen a large number of samples, spectroscopic and chromatographic systems are incorporating automation and robotics to do high-throughput analysis.

Thirdly, Data Analysis: Cutting-edge methods for deciphering large amounts of spectroscopic and chromatographic data, such as machine learning and artificial intelligence, are improving the quality of results.

4. Multimodal Approaches: By combining different spectroscopic or chromatographic techniques, scientists are able to conduct more in-depth chemical analysis and glean more nuanced insights from samples.

Summary: The Scientific Powerhouse Combo:

Analytical chemistry's guiding lights, spectroscopy and chromatography, shed light on the world's molecular complexities. These methods allow researchers in a wide variety of disciplines to probe, comprehend, and manipulate the properties of matter with greater ease and precision than ever before. Spectroscopy and chromatography are not just analytical tools but indispensable partners in the never-ending pursuit of scientific knowledge and technological advancement, whether that be in deciphering the structure of biomolecules, scrutinising environmental pollutants, or ensuring the quality of pharmaceuticals. As science and technology improve, we can expect to gain even deeper understandings of the chemical universe thanks to tools like spectroscopy and chromatography.

www.ingramcontent.com/pod-product-compliance
Lightning Source LLC
LaVergne TN
LVHW020442070526
838199LV00063B/4815